TOGETHER STRONG

I pray that this book enriches your life.

God bless!

Karen Erickson

TOGETHER STRONG

A JOURNEY OF FAITH, COMMUNITY CARE AND HUMAN STRUGGLES THROUGH CANCER

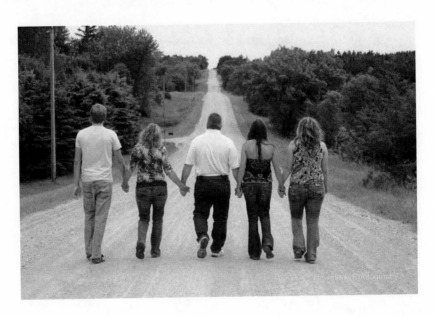

Karen Erickson

This is a true story. Only the first names of family and friends are used to protect them from the press and other related circumstances. Scripture quotations used in this book are from the Holy Bible.

This book was printed in the United States of America.

To order additional copies of this book, contact:
Xlibris Corporation
1-888-795-4274
www.Xlibris.com
Orders@Xlibris.com
97849

CONTENTS

I would like to dedicate this book
to everyone near and far who have supported us.

What Cancer Cannot Do

It Cannot . . .

Invade the soul

Suppress memories

Kill friendship

Destroy peace

Conquer the spirit

Shatter hope

Cripple love

Corrode faith

Steal eternal life

Silent courage

Karen, your daily messages were so beautiful—inspirational—and should be shared with the world.

—Sharon

Karen, I just wanted to let you know that I often reread your e-mails. When I get down or when I'm sad, I open one of your e-mails to lift me up. I don't know if you know it, but your e-mails are very inspirational. All the things your family has gone through and still how positive you have stayed and praying, praying, praying! I can totally see your face saying these words as you write them. You write like you are having a personal conversation with each of us on your e-mail chain. I can see your expressions and your arms waving around explaining every detail. :O) I needed a positive lift this morning and happened to come across one of your last e-mails. It must have been fate.

—Pam

Your strength and faith make us all reflect and give thanks for all we have been blessed with. God Bless.

—Paul

Everyone is put on earth for a purpose. Sometimes we know what our purpose is and other times we continue to search. I truly know that your family was here to bring many people closer to the Lord (which I know you have). Through the life you are living, you have truly taught others that the Lord is in control, and even through the ups and downs you are experiencing, your family has been a role model of what we are all suppose to be like on earth. Your family has touched so many lives and has taught all of us to count our blessings daily.

—Patty

Your writing is so heartfelt and honest. I hope that when Kevin is better and all this is behind you, you will write a book. It would have all the components of a good story. You hit every emotion, and your take on everything and everyone you meet is so refreshing. Your story shows the love of your faith, the love you have for each other, and the struggles in your life.

—Rita

Chapter 1

THE BEGINNING

It is so easy to take life for granted, and we all do this. Every minute, hour, and day are ours to live as we want or need. Life is busy, and it's easy to get distracted. Sometimes at the end of the day we remember and dwell on the mishaps more than the blessings that had happened.

There are so many blessings that each one of us has received from God. There are material blessings and also blessings that we can't see or touch. The smiles that touched our hearts, that we are alive, the moments, what we experienced, that we have emotions, and the memories that we made not only for us but for others too. Thank you, God, for the blessings that you have given me and that I am able to spread your good news through our trials in this book.

Unknowingly our lives started to change already in the spring of 2009, when my husband, Kevin, started noticing a muscle ache between his back blades. The aches never went away but instead fluctuated in pain intensity from time to time. We thought he was just getting older, and we continued on with life.

Our lives have always been very busy. There were not many nights that we were able to stay home as a family or by ourselves for a quiet evening for that matter. We were running to sporting events that the kids were involved in, gardening, working outside, getting together with friends and family, and volunteering at church, the local baseball tournament, at school, and in the community.

In September 2009, Kevin's pain got progressively worse. We thought the ache was worsened because he might have strained a muscle while working on the tractor, lifting something wrong, or simply pinched a nerve from sitting or sleeping in a wrong position. Kevin and I decided that it was time to go to the doctor.

He was able to see a chiropractor and physical therapist right away to try to relieve the immense pain he was enduring. Soon after, there was an opening for Kevin to see the medical doctor at his clinic that he's gone to since he was a child. Kevin's regular medical doctor wasn't available soon enough, so he saw someone else in the office on his visit. This doctor just told him to increase his Tylenol dose that he had already been taking. He was also given a prescription for a muscle relaxer. Kevin was instructed to continue the chiropractor and the physical therapy treatments. Kevin did everything he was told because he had confidence in the doctors at this time.

Dealing with pinched nerves and herniated disks myself, I couldn't understand how come he was reacting to pinched nerves or muscle aches like this. I have been in immense pain before but never carried on like this. I thought that I must just have a higher pain tolerance than him. Isn't this terrible for me to think like this? I felt bad feeling like this, but I just couldn't understand. I thought he was stronger or tougher than that.

Although Kevin was somewhat able to cover up his discomfort, he wanted to socialize with friends and family and tried to endure the pain and go on with life like normal. There were many times, however, that he just couldn't go out. We turned down house dinner parties and going to the maple syrup camp at the Doering home but did manage to have our annual holiday party because this always meant so much to Kevin.

By the second or third week in December, Kevin had no more mobility to turn his head. At times, he just groaned in frustration and confusion as to why the pain was so bad. The pain level brought him to tears many times, which is *very* uncommon for him.

A group of us had previously purchased tickets to go to a Christmas play in December. When the time came to go, Kevin felt too bad. His pain level was very high. He told me to go enjoy the play with our friends and that he would be okay. He didn't want me to miss the fun. I felt terrible going without him and leaving him home alone. I felt like I was abandoning him, but I knew he would be more comfortable at home. Here, he could sit in a chair that he knew would support his neck and not have to move his head at all.

TUESDAY, DECEMBER 22

Kevin had another therapy treatment today. After reviewing the treatment progress, the physical therapist told Kevin that his muscles should have been relaxed by this time. He didn't feel that he was helping Kevin anymore and he needed more intervention. At that time, Kevin told him that his neck was now numb and the pain was not tolerable at all. When this was said, the therapist told Kevin, "You need to see your medical doctor as soon as possible, today, right now! This isn't right. Something is wrong!"

I remember the call from Kevin after his visit like it was yesterday. I sensed some concern from Kevin, but I really wasn't alarmed or overly concerned because everyone had told us that it's a pinched nerve or muscle. After Kevin's call, I immediately called to schedule an appointment. We were able to get in for an appointment that same day, at 4:00 p.m., and Kevin's regular doctor was available this time. I was pleasantly surprised that we could get in so soon.

The doctor's office is about an hour away from our home. I remember feeling very stressed at this time. Kevin was in too much pain, so I drove. I wasn't used to driving in the cities. Not only that, but also there was road construction and rush hour had started. The traffic was terrible, and there were detours that we were unaware of. We were concerned that we would be late for our appointment but made it just in time.

At the appointment, the doctor concluded that Kevin needed stronger pain pills. We weren't satisfied with that prognosis at all. We requested an MRI. This was not only accomplished, but we were blessed with an MRI for six fifteen that *very same night*. We got scheduled to go to urgent care, which is just a few miles away from the clinic we were currently at. Kevin has claustrophobia and needed medication in order to relax during an MRI. A prescription was called in at the Walgreen's Pharmacy just around the corner from the doctor's office.

When I arrived at the pharmacy to pick it up, I was concerned. I noticed a line of customers waiting for their prescriptions already. I was worried that I wouldn't get the prescription soon enough. I couldn't help it. I paced back and forth until they called my name. We needed a certain amount of time for the drugs to react in order to be effective in helping Kevin. We were fortunate that we got this filled in such a timely manner. There were still some others waiting for their orders that were ahead of me, yet I still got the medicine we needed. The timing was perfect.

We arrived at urgent care and patiently waited in the office for Kevin's name to be called. Kevin and I were talking about our hopes for getting some answers. We felt some relief at this point. We felt that an MRI would tell it all, and we would be able to find out how to stop his pain. After the test, Kevin needed to recover for a little while. The doctors needed to make sure that the medication he took wore off before he left.

I remember sitting in the recovery room with him when the doctor came in and said, "I have some bad news." I held my breath as I'm sure Kevin did too, along with disbelief that there would even be anything seriously wrong or bad to report. The doctor said, "The MRI showed a shadow on Kevin's vertebrae that is probably a large tumor. We probably will need emergency surgery to remove it and it may be cancerous." We were stunned. The doctors even showed us the shadow as we looked at the x-ray. It was so big! The doctors were concerned that it had wrapped around the vertebrae but weren't positive of the degree. They said we needed more testing.

I still remember the feeling of emptiness and hopelessness as Kevin and I looked at each other in disbelief. Not even saying a word, we both cried silently, with tears running down our faces, just looking at each other. We didn't say anything for what seemed like eternity. I went over to Kevin and hugged him, trying to embrace him with firmness as to comfort him. How could this be? Kevin never smoked, his family history didn't include this disease, he's a healthy man . . . So many thoughts were going through our minds at this time. How could I have been so insensitive as to think that Kevin couldn't endure nerve or muscle pain when the whole time it was *this*! I was numb. If only we would have known. Why did we wait to ask for an MRI?

They told us that we were very fortunate to be in doctor's care that very moment because it was very possible that he would have died from this by the weekend. The tumor may have already eaten the bone used to support his spine, and it's possible that the nerves could have pinched off his breathing.

We were then told to go immediately to North Memorial emergency using *extreme caution*. Being as it was winter, if Kevin would slip, get a whiplash, or fall, he could break his neck. The medical staff were very concerned about this and put a temporary brace on Kevin to help support his neck. We all believed that the fastest and safest way to get Kevin to the emergency room was for me to drive him myself. The ambulance needed time to travel to get where we were to get Kevin, and we didn't have time to wait. We also were told that the ride in the ambulance could be very bumpy, and we didn't need any jerking of his head at the time.

The doctors brought Kevin to the car in a wheelchair for me. They told me that they called the emergency room already, letting them know we're on our way. I was comforted to hear that there would be someone waiting for us at the emergency entrance with a wheelchair to get Kevin when we arrive.

I'm not familiar driving in the cities at all, especially at night, in winter, and in these circumstances. Kevin patiently guided me as to which roads to turn onto in order to get where we needed to be. Once we were there, they were ready for him just like we were told and rushed him in the emergency center while I parked the car. Once I made it to the emergency entrance, I was greeted by an employee to take me to a waiting area until I could see Kevin. I was frantic, along with so many things going through my mind. I can't even imagine what Kevin was thinking of but am sure that he wanted me by his side the whole time.

While the doctors were examining him, I called the kids. I told them that Kevin needed more testing but that they found what was causing his pain. I informed them that this was serious and possibly cancer. They were all very concerned and upset, of course. I reassured them that I would keep them informed with everything, they could trust me, and I would be honest with them. They would be the first ones I call with any new information. I then called our families, informing them the severity of this neck pain.

This was so upsetting for everyone! What a shock! They were also in disbelief and were very concerned about all of us. At this time, I felt this is all a blur. It's like I couldn't believe this is true. Is this a dream? Is this really happening? Each phone call I made was like I needed to keep repeating what was going on so I could believe that it truly was happening to us.

The doctors met with Kevin and me and told us that he would need to go to the hospital for more testing and surgery to remove this tumor. My family and Kevin wanted me to go home for the night to be with the kids and make a plan for the upcoming days ahead. As long as there was nothing more going to happen that night, I could come back to be with Kevin in the morning. I didn't want to leave, but Kevin insisted that I was needed at home too and he would be fine without me.

I will never forget the drive home. I was crying, praying in silence, praying out loud, planning on how I'm going to tell the kids the details that were known at this time. Thinking, planning, organizing, and repeating this over and over again in my mind to rethink my decisions. It was only a little over an hour's drive to get home, but it seemed like it took forever.

It was late when I got home, but the kids waited up for me. I was able to spend time with them, explaining what we knew at this time. There were a lot of tears and confusion, but we agreed to pull together and work together during this difficult time. We planned a strategy of who will do the chores and discussed the need of communication between us all. We needed to make sure that everyone got where they needed to be when I'm not home.

Now remember that all of this took place in one day/night. I know God was there for us from the start of this day. This is proven by the necessity that was given for Kevin and the appointment openings that were made readily available for us at this time already. This whole string of events in which we were able to get in to see the doctors so quickly and get some results and the schedules in place really amazed me.

Wednesday, December 23

As soon as I got up in the morning, I made sure the kids were off to school and the chores were done. Then I was on my way back to North Memorial to be by Kevin's side.

Pastor Joel came to the ICU and prayed with me over Kevin. We were focused on prayer and faith for healing. He read and discussed the following Bible verse with us. Philippians 4:4 says, "Rejoice in the Lord always. I will say it again: Rejoice! Let your gentleness be evident to all. The Lord is near. Do not be anxious about anything, but in everything, by prayer and petition, with thanksgiving, present your requests to God. And the peace of God, which passes all understanding, will guard your hearts and your minds in Christ Jesus."

The definition for *anxious* is being uneasy, fearful, or worried. In other words, Joel said, "Don't worry about anything. When someone worries, they are leaving room for the Devil to work his way in. Trust in the Lord completely." God has plans for us all. Worrying about the unknown or future isn't going to help us. It's easy to say, but we all need to put our faith in our Father in Heaven. Joel also prayed for me and the family that we would be comforted and given peace. Both Kevin and I appreciated his visit very much.

A CT scan was taken and read by a neurology specialist. I prayed that we would have some answers today. The results from the CT scan showed a tumor that ate away his C2 vertebrae and some of his C3 vertebrae and also was wrapped in front of his spine. North Memorial hospital wasn't equipped for the required surgery. We were told that Kevin would be transferred tomorrow to Abbott NW Hospital for emergency surgery.

Oh, my God! What just happened? They didn't say it was cancer, just a tumor that needs to be removed NOW. We both are trying to concentrate on Joel's message and keep the faith.

I am so very thankful that my sister, Penny, insisted on coming up to be with me tonight. Her son, Jeff, lives only a couple of miles away from this hospital. After spending some time with Kevin, we were able to go to his house to spend the night. This way, I wouldn't have to do a ton of driving or stay overnight at a hotel. The weather was getting really bad too. We are getting a snowstorm and I'm better off staying up here.

Penny, Jeff, and his roommate, Brant, tried to make it as comfortable as possible for me. They tried not to talk too much about the situation, but it was healing for me to inform them of what all transpired. We got take-out food, and after supper, we visited and made plans for the days ahead. There was so much to plan. There was so much unknown at the time. I talk a lot anyway, but when I'm nervous, at times I talk even more. It's like a nervous talk or something. I tried to relax as best as I could, and when we went to bed. I just relaxed and prayed to God for help over and over and over again.

Chapter 2

SURGERY

THURSDAY, DECEMBER 24

Today is Christmas Eve, and everything went as we had planned. It was really cold and had snowed a lot during the night. Jeff cleared the snow off Penny's truck and shoveled around it so we could get out. Before we left, Jeff assured me that he would take care of our truck and its contents. By leaving the truck at his home, we wouldn't need to be concerned of theft or vandalism to the truck in the parking garage at the hospital ramp and I wouldn't need to pay for parking.

While Kevin was being transferred, Penny drove me to Abbott Hospital. Travel was terrible, and we needed to take our time because the roads were very icy. We got to the hospital early in the day and found our way to the eighth floor, where Kevin was. It was so nice to see him, and I was glad that I could be there for him. He looked really scared but seemed to be relieved to see me. Kevin commented on the bumpy ambulance ride he had, "It was terrible. I couldn't wait for it to end."

The doctors came in the room and gave us notice as to when they would need to get Kevin to prepare him for surgery. Kevin and I were given some alone time before the doctors came to take him away. I remember feeling helpless and wishing that our hug and kiss would last forever. I didn't want to let him go. I was afraid that he wouldn't come back to me. I didn't want him to leave with the doctors, even though I knew he needed to in order to stay alive.

While they were prepping Kevin for surgery, Penny and I went to a Christmas Eve service at the chapel in the hospital. We really didn't like the sermon and/or the way it was presented at all. We ignored the minister, and each of us just spent time with the Lord in prayer. We were still in the House of God and felt his presence. After this, we were directed to the specific waiting room where we needed to be. This way, the doctor would be able to locate us after surgery was completed to go over the surgery.

While waiting for the surgery to be over, Penny helped me understand some important mail and paperwork Kevin was working on. He brought it with him to the doctor appointment to finish. This was really unusual for him to do, so I thought that it was important and needed immediate attention. He also had our bills that were due along with him. She helped me with this too because I had a hard time focusing and paying attention to detail. She took whatever I needed mailed and said she'd get the business papers taken to the office where they needed to be. This was a huge lift off of my shoulders.

The phone calls were never ending during this time. I understood that everyone just needed to know what was happening and they were also showing me support during this time.

After a number of hours of operating, Dr. Garner came to tell me that the surgery was a success. He explained it like this to us: "The doctor's decided to take a donor bone to replace the vertebrae instead of using a bone from Kevin. The reason for this is because they didn't want to make another incision anywhere on Kevin's body to extract any bone. If they would have, that would just be another opening that could get infected. They felt this was the safer thing to do. The donor bone was used to replace the C2 vertebrae and repair the C3 vertebrae. The doctor's fused C1 vertebrae to the C2 vertebrae and the C1 vertebrae to the C3 vertebrae."

At this time, we were still waiting on the results of the testing to find out if it is cancer or not. If it is cancer, we will find out what treatment will kill it. If it is not cancer, after Kevin is healed from this surgery, they will do another surgery to remove the remaining tumor in front of his spine. They couldn't do this at this time because there was no way to support Kevin's neck, being as they just replaced and repaired the damage that was done. There is no strength in the spine yet for another surgery. Kevin was kept in the ICU at this time due to his blood pressure and oxygen levels.

There was a big snowstorm during this time, and safe travel was a concern for our kids. Being as it is Christmas Eve and we will not be home, I needed to make sure they will be celebrating Christ's birth safely.

I asked Kevin's brother-in-law to clear the driveway of snow on the farm and make sure the dogs get to Sally's kennel. This way, the kids wouldn't need to worry about coming home to take care of them. I also asked if he and his wife, Nancy, Kevin's sister, would take the kids to their home for a family Christmas celebration for Christmas Eve and Christmas day. I asked for them to make sure the kids stay at their home and not go to other family member's homes due to the poor travel conditions. We have enough to worry about much less they get in an accident or have difficulties.

There were stresses put on the kids due to other family members wanting them for the Christmas holiday that day. Everyone just wanted to help, but I knew I could count on Nancy to take care of those stresses for them and us. Christmas was really different for all of us this year. We missed the kids, but Kevin and I were pretty calm. We were thinking that the majority of the problem of the tumor is over with, and we are at peace with what all transpired. We had hopes of turning the corner.

I remember being hungry in the evening and telling Kevin that I was going to get something to eat and take a break. I went to McDonald's that was located in the hospital and got chicken nuggets, fries, and a chocolate shake. I felt I deserved the shake today. I went to the entrance of the hospital and sat on a couch with my meal, admiring the beautiful decorations and the beautiful music that the player piano made.

As I ate my food, I gave thanks to God our Father for bringing Kevin out of the surgery back to the kids and me. I was thankful for the wisdom of the doctors and asked for continued healing. I just loved this time alone to think and relax. I really appreciated and felt comforted from the soft, gentle music that was echoing in the entire lobby entrance where I was seated. Remarkably, I remember feeling such peace at this time. The huge Christmas tree that was standing in front of me was so very stunning, with many colors and lights. The lights made me feel the brightness of life and the magnificence of miracles and faith. Everything was so peaceful and quiet.

I felt very sad not being with my children, but understood that they couldn't be here. I knew that they were celebrating Christmas with family and cousins their own age, hoping they have fun and, at the same time, hopeful that this will occupy their minds and keep them from constantly thinking about what's happening.

The nurses told me that I was supposed to stay at an adjoining hotel during the evening. I told them that I promised Kevin that I wouldn't step one foot out of this hospital so I wouldn't go. I didn't want to put any more stress on Kevin at this time. He always worries about me getting lost due to my health conditions and previous amnesia incidents. Once I gave my reasons, the nurses allowed me to stay in the family waiting area on the condition that I don't take a private family room for more than three hours. I was able to pull two chairs together, laid my head down, and put another chair in front of me to support my knees. I got real used to this. Besides, who could sleep anyway. I constantly looked in on Kevin and walked the halls.

Friday, December 25

It's Christmas today. I was able to be with Kevin in the ICU room this morning when he woke up. The doctor came in to let us know that they needed to and were working on finding the source of this tumor and the results will hopefully come next week. Another CT scan of Kevin's neck was done, and the results are also unknown at this time. Kevin was moved out of the ICU later in the day, and we were both able to stay together in a hospital room. This was the same floor as before, so we were kind of familiar as to where everything was.

We have already been called by some friends wanting to help with meals for the kids. I had some meals already prepared in the freezer and was hoping to be home early next week, so I only needed one or two for now.

Kevin has been very emotional whenever a family member or special friend called. He also has a difficult time holding in his tears whenever someone leaves. I have never seen him like this before. I'm sure that he is aware of how blessed he is to be alive and is so thankful that he sheds tears of joy, love, and happiness.

Kevin told me that I needed to purchase him a laptop computer so he can work from wherever he is.

SATURDAY, DECEMBER 26
(update typed MONDAY, DECEMBER 28, 4:35 A.M.)

A gentleman from the brace company came to fit a new brace on Kevin. This brace has more support and will be more comfortable for long-term wear. He showed both of us how to properly fit this on Kevin. At this time, he also went over the use and care instructions with us. It is important for me to keep it cleaned properly.

Everything seemed to be going well. We were comfortable and had been enjoying each other's company. The doctors came in to talk to us. We were pleasantly surprised when they told us that it's possible that we would be going home as soon as two to four days from now. Wow, how far medicine has come. Years ago, this would never have happened. This was such a serious surgery!

When Alan and Penny came to visit us, they brought our truck to the hospital. This way, we could go home right away as soon as Kevin was released in a few days.

Kevin enjoyed the day, but it really made him tired. He showed off his neck brace with our visitors. John and Nancy, Al and Dede, Scott and Brenda and Mike all came to give Kevin support. I was able to sleep on the couch in the same room as Kevin that night, which was really nice for both of us. I was really tired too, being as I didn't get much sleep the night before. I was looking forward to the rest.

Chapter 3

REACTION AND COMPLICATIONS

This was a new day for us. We were really excited with the news we received yesterday of possibly coming home soon. I remember overhearing the doctor's talk among themselves during the midmorning rounds. They were happy with how Kevin was recovering from the surgery so they had removed the pain meds that they had been giving him.

By midafternoon, Kevin started getting agitated. He has claustrophobia, and he had told me around 5:00 p.m. that he felt like everything was closing in on him. I tried to make him comfortable and occupy his time to help with his anxiousness. We communicated this all to the doctors and explained again of the claustrophobia he has experienced in the past. They gave Kevin some medication to help him relax. I could tell that the medicine he was given really wasn't helping him at all. He was now feeling like he needed to get out of the room and felt closed in.

We were hoping that the reason for this agitation was that the medicine just didn't kick in yet. Kevin tried to be content and patient while watching TV and visiting with me. When I went to sleep on the couch that night, Kevin started acting really strange. I didn't really think anything of it at the time; I just laughed and went to bed on the couch.

A short time later, Kevin called for me, and I stood up to see what he wanted. He just said, "Hey! You have four eyes!" I thought that' was weird, but whatever. I laid back down on the couch, and all of a sudden all *hell* broke loose!

To put it mildly, Kevin wasn't acting like himself at all! He was very agitated and had tried to get out of bed. He isn't supposed to get out of bed alone. He was to have his head supported and get assistance to move. He didn't make any sense of what he was saying. He kept mumbling and yelling. He got mad at me because I was trying to keep him in bed and protect his neck. He had one thing on his mind, and he was determined to do it.

His neck was very weak yet at this point. He was told that he needed to stay put for maximum neck support. I was so concerned that his neck was going to break with all of his movement at this point already. When I wasn't able to calm him down anymore or keep him lying down, I called for a nurse to help me get him back in bed.

The nurse checked to see what medications they had already administered to him at that time and made adjustments as they felt was needed. I thought the incident was all over. I was relieved that the nurse came in and addressed the problem. I thought that as soon as the medicine took hold, we could both get some much-needed rest. I went back to bed, but it wasn't long after that when he got upset again! I tried really hard to contain him, but I couldn't settle him down. I needed to call for the nurse to help me again.

I was given permission to take Kevin for strolls from time to time with the wheelchair in hopes to reduce his anxiousness. I thought it would make the time fly faster for him and give him some space. I pushed him to various rooms on the eighth floor of the hospital, which overlooked the city. I stayed positive for him and showed him the beautiful lights and stars. I carried on conversations as best I could without letting him know that I was scared as to what was happening to him.

Our hopes that these trips out and about would satisfy his agitation were short lived. Soon his attention for this went awry too, and I was not able to keep his concentration. I couldn't even manage to keep him seated in the wheelchair either anymore. It was a struggle, but I managed to get him back to his room while asking for help on the way. I quit trying to take him for walks at this time. His agitation went on all night long. The incidents became much more often, and he became angrier and stronger. Soon we needed to have two nurses help me and then three.

Sometimes the nurses increased the medications; sometimes they changed the medicines. Other times, they decreased one and added another medication when we couldn't control him. I couldn't keep track of what they were doing anymore. As you all know, Kevin had a neck brace that was imperative that he wore to support his neck. It was a *very* snug brace that supported his head, snuggling his neck, and it rested on his shoulders. Kevin was able to rest his chin on it for support.

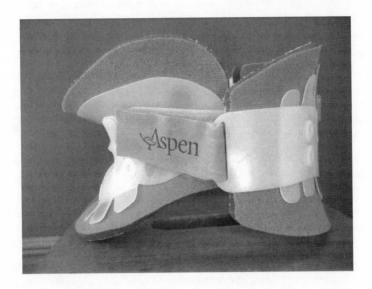

Neither doctors nor I could even begin to imagine how in the world Kevin was able to push this brace off his head. Not only once but two or three times. I watched him! He didn't even turn his head to weasel his way out of it. I couldn't believe it! We were all concerned that he was going to pull apart the fusion, become paralyzed, or need another surgery. He continuously was struggling to pull out his catheter and medicine tubes too! I lost track of how many times they needed to reinsert the medicine needle in his arm.

The nurses didn't know what else to do for Kevin other than reevaluate his medicines and increase or change them according to his reactions. I recall a couple of times when they couldn't believe how strong the medicines were that they had given him and he was still able to struggle. They would say, "Oh my God, he is a *very strong* man. I can't believe it!"

After awhile, which seemed like forever, the staff felt that it was safer to restrain his arms so he wouldn't be able to take out any needles, get out of bed, or tear his catheter out. Why didn't any of us think of that before this? It took a while, but after the restraints were on securely, the medical staff had left the room. They were confident that the incidences were over. Kevin called me over to his bedside. I rushed to him and felt devastated to see him so helpless. I touched his arm and tried to reassure him that he was going to be all right.

He then asked me to release the restraints. I, of course, gave him good reasons why I couldn't. He got frustrated with me. I felt bad that I couldn't but proceeded to turn around and go back to the couch to try to get some sleep.

As soon as I got comfortable, Kevin asked for me to come to his bedside again. This time, he asked me to cut him loose, and I refused. This made him *really* mad. All of a sudden, his left leg swung over his right hip and he pushed me with such force that

I flew five to six feet back into the bookcase. Never underestimate a patient who knows what they want, especially when they are drugged up.

Not only was he determined, but also he is smart. With kicks of his legs, Kevin was able to bounce his butt downward on the bed. This allowed his elbows and shoulders closer to the restraints, loosening them so he could try to get freed, pulled his medicine needle out again, and tried to get his catheter out. I called for help again, and the nursing staff gave him more drugs. They realigned him to the bed by pulling him up onto the bed with the bed sheet. They would talk to him calmly, and as soon as we thought progress was happening, it started over again.

The doctors asked me about the alcohol intake Kevin currently had on a weekly or daily basis. I told them that Kevin only social drinks and that I know he doesn't have an alcohol problem for sure. They continued to ask me for the number of drinks, and I answered if we have any, he has one to two drinks per occasion. I was upset with the assumption the doctors had because they weren't even considering anything else to be the cause at this time. I just knew there was something wrong and that it wasn't alcohol related. They told me that they were going to treat Kevin as if he is having alcohol withdrawals because they don't have any reason to believe that this isn't the case.

I don't know why this upset me so much, but it did. The episodes became longer and longer and the amount of time between them was shorter and shorter until there was no break in the episodes at all. It came to the point where there needed to be about six nurses trying to keep Kevin down in the bed. Two of the nurses were larger, stronger men that had been in and out of the room the entire night, helping when needed. They were all trained for this type of thing.

The nurses ended up calling for 2 security officers. They needed more help in restraining Kevin because at this point, six of them were not enough. It's like he was possessed. When security came, they were concerned because they were told that Kevin kicked someone. They didn't know who it was, so when they asked I said, "It was me and I am his wife and this isn't the way my husband acts."

This time, they also restrained Kevin's legs. Why didn't any of us think of that before either? They gave him more relaxant drugs and had asked me to leave the room. They could see that I was of no help to them or Kevin at this point anymore. They also didn't feel it was necessary for me to see him go through this. It isn't healthy or good for me.

I went to the waiting room to pray and call some family members, explaining what was going on. Nobody could understand. The family was actually angry that the doctors were treating this as Kevin having an alcoholic reaction. I called my friend, Judy, who is a nurse also and asked her if one to two drinks could affect someone like this and her answer didn't make me feel any better at all. The answer was yes it could.

First of all, this would mean that Kevin is an alcoholic, which means a long-term fix and which means I also am probably an alcoholic because I have one or two drinks some nights with him also. I still didn't believe this was the case, and we just need to wait it out. This means no more drinking for either of us if this is true, and after this is done, I definitely will want a drink.

I then started pacing the halls of the hospital floor, thinking, trying to understand, and crying in disbelief. As I started down the hall where his room was, I could hear him struggling in bed. It was a terrible sound to hear. The sound of the bed mattress pushing the bed frame from him, pushing his body back and forth; his legs kicking up and down as high as they would go and hitting the bed; the restraints being pulled tightly and shaking the side bars on the bed frame. As I reached his room, I could see in only a little bit because they had the door partially closed. I glanced through the small opening as I was walking. I didn't want him to hear or see that I was there. I didn't want him to call for me. He was struggling so much! My heart was broken just to see this and realized that seeing it is even worse than hearing it.

I heard him yelling, screaming, and then mumbling words that didn't make any sense at all. It was easy to see that he was extremely mad and angry because nobody would come to his aid when he called for them. I wanted to go in and try to comfort him but was too exhausted by this time and left him alone.

Kevin had to be physically exhausted because of all he has been through already. Somehow he was still able to muster up the strength to try to yank the arm and leg restraints off of the bed so he could escape. He tried over and over and over again but never succeeded.

Soon the nurses came and pulled the curtain so his voice wouldn't carry so far down the hall, and he would also then have less noise distraction himself. They wanted him to rest if at all possible. I went to the waiting room and waited for the staff to come talk to me about Kevin and what was going on.

There was a computer that was available for me to use. I felt the need to let others know what has been happening. I felt that the more people know, the more prayers will be said. I wrote my first e-mail to a large list of family and friends. This e-mail explained *very* briefly of everything that had happened. This night seemed to go on forever. I didn't sleep at all. All I could do was pray, cry, pace the halls, and wait. I waited for the doctors to come and tell me that I could go back in the room to be with Kevin. That never happened. My heart was broken! It was *really* a long night.

MONDAY, DECEMBER 28, 11:30 P.M.

In the afternoon, the nurses told me to go home because I wasn't doing any good being at the hospital anymore. It was really hard to leave. I felt like I was abandoning him. What do I tell the kids when I get home? How do I give them hope?

It was really hard not to think about Kevin and the situation at hand throughout the entire day. I tried to keep myself very occupied. I called the hospital from time to time to check on him throughout the day and evening. Each time I spoke with the nurse in charge of Kevin, I was told that there was no change.

In the early evening, the staff felt they couldn't restrain him from hurting himself or others any longer, so they sent him back to the intensive care unit. In the ICU, they put Kevin in a drug-induced coma, along with a respirator and oxygen to keep him quiet. This is the best place for him right now because they can keep a more constant watch on him. His blood pressure has been high a lot also the last few days, and this also needed to be monitored closer. Right now, the doctors want me to stay home and call back tomorrow. They will let me know when they want me to meet with them to discuss the issues at hand.

I am very thankful to the medical staff. They wouldn't allow visitors, but they allowed our minister in to be with Kevin. Joel and his wife, Mary Lou, went to see Kevin in the ICU to pray again. After the visit, they called me to tell me that he looked very peaceful and good. I felt very sad that I wasn't among them during their visit. I had a need to touch him, talk to him, make him feel secure that he was with me, feel the warmth of his hand, and kiss him. Being as that was not the case, I still was comforted by this call. It's like Mary Lou was my eyes and my hands as they touched him in prayer.

In the evening, I asked the kids if they wanted to open one Christmas present. They decided on opening a gift they received from each other. They wanted to save the rest for when Kevin would be home. It just wasn't the same. There wasn't the usual excitement or laughter that went along with opening presents. It was still nice. Kevin was missing, and it was not the same for any of us.

I am very grateful but not surprised with the outpour of support and prayers from friends and family. I truly know that prayer is the way to recovery from *every* situation in life, and this is no exception.

Everything that has happened to us during this situation has been a blessing from God. If Kevin hadn't had his neck pain, we wouldn't have known that he had a tumor. This is wonderful that we were able to catch this before it was too late. We put Kevin at the foot of the cross and prayed that he would stay free of infections, pneumonia, cancer, and injury to the operated area and that he would stay strong and confident in God during this time. Kevin is usually the rock, and it is now our turn. We will be Kevin's rock, keeping positive that he is in God's hands.

I was concerned that friends and family would need to have ongoing accurate information. I needed everyone to know the truth, not gossip. E-mail updates will let everyone know what to pray for and eliminate many calls to me asking for details. At this time, I didn't even want to think about keeping an e-mail list updated, adding names and correcting addresses. I need to concentrate on Kevin and the kids only. I asked our good friends Patti and Al if they would be the hosts of my "Kevin update" e-mails. Being as I sent an e-mail last night, they had the core list of addresses already.

I continued sending daily e-mails to our friends Patti and Al. When Al, Patti, or I would hear of anyone that wanted to be included in the updates, we would communicate and Al and Patti would each update their lists. They did a wonderful job including so many addresses. There also were contacts from Norwood, Eden Prairie, Maple Lake,

South Haven, and Howard Lake that also decided to be hosts of additional groups of people. They would forward the e-mails that they already received from Patti or Al to their list of addresses.

My daughter, Stephanie, made a folder on the computer titled "Kevin's love prayers." All of the e-mails of prayers, notes, and well wishes that are being sent our way for Kevin will get put in there for him to read when he comes out of this.

TUESDAY, DECEMBER 29, 10:11 P.M.

I called the hospital as soon as I got up for the day. I was told that Kevin is still sedated but resting very well. His reflexes are working and oxygen level is good. He will be sedated again today, possibly undergoing another CT scan to make sure that he didn't reinjure his neck during the difficulty and the struggles he has endured the last couple of days. CT scans are tough on Kevin, so it's good to do this when he is sedated.

I am praying for the doctor to call me today. As soon as they do, I will e-mail everyone. Everything is going well here at home. I need to keep life with as much normalcy as possible for the kids. Life does seem to go on, even if it's not easy or convenient at the time.

Many people have called and offered their help in any way possible. I started a list for the kids and me to refer to. On this list are people's names and their phone numbers that we can call. Next to that, I wrote down what they are willing to help with. Some want to help with rides; with meals; plow the snow on the yard, in the dry lots, and on the road; clean the house; and do other miscellaneous things. I kept a copy of this list with me when I was away and put one on the refrigerator at home for the kids to refer to when they needed anything.

I have volunteered a lot in the past and know from experience how good it feels to give to others. It's very comforting to feel like you've made a difference for someone by helping in any way, when one doesn't know what to say or do, to make life easier for them. It's also wonderful that you are able to give them something to be thankful for and to show God's love. I found out that it's much harder to receive help than it is to give it. Is it pride? Is it just being stubborn? Is it because I feel that we don't deserve it?

I thought about this and realized that Kevin's sickness affects more than our families, children, and me. It also affects our friends and communities. I know that people offer to help because they want to. By asking and accepting help from others, not only will it help the kids, Kevin, and I, but also it will help them too.

I was called by Jamie from our church. She was in charge of making sure that food and meal situations were taken care of for families of the sick or injured people in our congregation. It was nice to be able to call her among others who have volunteered to donate meals when needed. Between the church, friends, family, and the community, we never had to worry about the kids or me going hungry.

Being as I couldn't help Kevin at the hospital right now, I tried to think of things that I could do that would help Kevin when he comes back home. This helped me look toward the future. Will he be stressed out to see the things that need to be done around the house? He still won't be able to do most of them when he comes home due to his brace and restrictions.

The windows in our house are pretty bad. We had purchased some pleated blinds in the fall to help with the drafty windows. We also thought these blinds would help reduce the heating bill. Kevin had intended on installing the blinds in both of the girl's bedrooms and Tony's bedroom before winter. Due to his neck pain and mobility problems, he wasn't able to put them up. We both kept saying that it will get done as soon as his neck felt better. Well, that day never came.

Our neighbor Phil is what I call a handyman at trade. He enjoys fixing, building things, and simply doing things for others. He stopped by today and offered me his help. I knew I couldn't do this myself so I asked him to install the blinds for us. Not only did he do this for us, but also he did a perfect job. The kids and I were so happy that he did this for us. I know that Kevin will be relieved that this was done when he comes home.

I am thankful that Kevin is where he is right now because this could have really been tragic had we waited or not been able to get in to see the doctor when we did. I am also thankful for the wonderful network of friends and family to keep us strong.

The doctor called later today. I can see Kevin in the morning. Hopefully the doctors will be able to answer some questions for us.

Before I went to bed, I called the ICU again and asked the nurse on call to pray over Kevin for me.

I received the following prayer from a dear friend of mine, reminding us of our friendship and the support given:

I thought of you so much today
I went to God in prayer,
To ask Him to watch over you
And show you that I care.
My prayer for you was not for rewards
That you could touch or feel,
But true rewards for happiness
That are so very real.
Like love and understanding
In all the things you do,
And guidance when you need it most
To see your troubles through.
I asked Him for good health for you
So your future could be bright,
And faith to accept life's challenges
And the courage to do what's right.
I gave thanks to Him
For granting my prayer

To bring you peace and love.
May you feel the warmth in your life
With God's blessings from above

WEDNESDAY, DECEMBER 30

The doctors had planned on meeting with me this morning to update me on Kevin's well-being. I felt I needed to have another set of ears to help me remember what the doctors all said to me, so I asked Kevin's brother, Lester to come too. Lester, met me in Rockford, and we drove to the hospital together.

Lester suggested that I bring a tablet of paper and pen with me to the future doctor meetings. This way, I can write down the facts that are given us. Sometimes it's easier to remember when I reread them. I can also write down any questions that I have for the doctors in between appointments so I won't forget them and have them handy the next time we meet.

When we arrived, it was so very hard to see Kevin pinned down. He was still tied to the bed at this time because he has times of agitation and struggles yet. Not only that, but he also had tubes running every which way you could even imagine. They needed to keep him still so he wouldn't bother the tubes. Kevin is in need of complete rest, and I was asked again by the medical staff for no visitation from *anyone*.

The doctors didn't have answers to anything at this time. The nursing staff thinks that it's possible that Kevin is irritated partially because of the breathing tube being in and down his throat. Because of this, they tried a different type of sedation medicine today in hopes to try to wean him off of the ventilator. This *didn't work*!

As long as I was there, the nurses allowed me to be with Kevin for a while alone. I was able to be near him, touching him, talking to him, and reassuring him. It felt so good to have this time together even if it was just for a short while. I was hoping that I would help him to relax and feel comforted, but instead, he just got more agitated. I felt terrible! I couldn't understand why he got upset with me there again. The nurses asked me to leave the room because they all had to rush in there to settle him down and they needed all the room that was available.

What is happening! I thought. Why is this happening? This isn't like my husband! I mean, I'm his wife! Doesn't Kevin want me there? Doesn't he love me anymore? Does he even know what's going on? Can't he hear me? Why is he acting like this? What did I do to him? Did I say something wrong? I'm very hurt that I can't help him and calm him. I feel helpless!

We need to remember that the reason for the sedation is to protect the airway and the surgical area by keeping him calm.

I felt like I needed to be with Kevin through this trial, but instead I was told to go home again. They told me to call from time to time if I wanted and come back tomorrow. On the way home, I called the kids and informed them of what news I had received. We then planned on a time later on in the day when we could get together as a family and do something together.

I wanted to eliminate making so many phone calls and spending so much time and energy by calling each person in the family. I knew I needed a plan. I decided that the kids are the first to be updated with Kevin's progress. Once they are informed, I will inform family. I decided to only call one person in my family and one of Kevin's siblings. I asked each of them to pass the information I gave them at the time to the rest of the family. I took turns with whom I called each time in case they had any additional questions that they didn't get answered before. All of their names are also on the e-mail update list, so if they didn't understand fully, they would be able to read that also.

After I have completed those calls, I will then do an update e-mail to Al and Patti. They will in turn pass it forward to others who want to be in the loop. By this time, already the e-mail list had grown quite large. Updates have been going all over Minnesota to Colorado to Florida and who knows where else this news was traveling. Just think of all of the prayers that are coming Kevin's way!

Later on in the day, Karen, who is the youth director of our church, called. She asked if we would like her to come over to pray with us. We all agreed that we needed her to come to visit with us at home. Not only did she graciously do this, but also she brought each one of us a special gift. She gave Tony, Kaylee, Stephanie, and me a journal book. She felt that it would be helpful for us to write our feelings and thoughts on paper. She also gave me a CD to take to the hospital for Kevin. She was hoping that if the nurses would play this CD in Kevin's room, it would calm and relax him. Kevin isn't into music, but I said, "It's worth a shot."

Before I went to bed, I called the ICU and asked for updates. I ended my call again by asking the nurse if she could put her hand on Kevin in prayer, which they were always more than happy to do for us.

THURSDAY, DECEMBER 31, 11:28 P.M.

We wish each and every one of you a very blessed New Year. Lester, Kevin's brother, met me in Rockford again this morning and drove me to the hospital. We were to meet with the ICU nurse and the radiologist. I was proud to show Lester that I had remembered my tablet and pen for notes at the appointment. When we met with the doctors I needed to let them know of my traumatic brain injury. I explained how I will need to write down facts and ask many questions so I'm clear as to what they are saying. I asked them to please be patient with me. We were very pleased with the information we received and the quality of care Kevin has been receiving.

We were told that today, they are going to try a different medication that will go into the feeding tube to help calm him down. I tried the CD Karen gave me, but he didn't seem to like it. I will give it to someone else who can use it.

The doctor's also did an EEG today, and the neurological surgeon and the neurologist will look at the readings to try to eliminate the unknown causes for agitation. They will consider doing another MRI or CT scan if necessary. Tomorrow, they will try to start dropping sedation levels gradually to see if they can calmly get him alert.

Kevin's currently on blood thinner to keep the blood from clotting, and they will hopefully start to give him diuretics to help relieve the swelling that has occurred. His tongue is swollen from the respirator and his wrists and ankles are also swollen from the restraints. This is all normal due to being in the bed for this period of time. The restraints will need to stay on no matter what due to the safety issue for him and others.

The doctors don't feel they can wait any longer to continue care for Kevin's tumor, so radiation will be done by Monday for sure, whether he is sedated or not. They will do radiation on C1, C2, C3, and C4 to kill the tumor. They still don't know at this time if the tumor is cancerous or not, but they know that it's not good having it there anymore. The good news is that while sedated, things that are going well are Kevin's nutrition and the neurologic exam results. His blood pressure is also good, and he is very stable at this time. Kevin is in the right place, and with all of our prayers, he hopefully will be recovering soon.

I was afraid that the nurses were going to tell me that they didn't want me to be in the room with Kevin again due to the agitation he had in recent visits. I reassured them that I will be good, in hopes that they would let me try to visit again. You see, the nurses think that having me in the room and the sound of my voice gets Kevin anxious, upset, worried, etc. They did, however, allow me to visit with him today, and it definitely went better than yesterday. I tried not to talk too much to Kevin, which was hard for me to do. So much has happened that I wanted to share with him. I also needed to use a soft voice, which I found very hard to do also. I was so excited to see him, touch him, and be with him.

The doctor's are currently allowing a few visitations from family only.

On the way back from the hospital, I called Kevin's siblings and asked them and whoever else wanted to meet me at the office for a family meeting. Lester dropped me off at my truck and went to the office ahead of me. On the way to the office, I prayed to God, asking him to keep me strong and be with me during the meeting. One of my weaknesses due to my brain injury is difficulty with explanations; I have a hard time keeping up when topics change and staying focused as to what I was saying so the facts could be relayed correctly. I needed to do all of these in order to be able to answer any of the questions they had.

When I arrived at work, everybody was there in Kevin's office already. They were anxiously and cautiously waiting for the news. I knew that I needed to be strong at this time. I wanted to reassure them all that everything would be all right. I also needed them to know that I could handle this and to trust me that I will keep them up to date with any test results. I wanted them to know that I will make good decisions and take care of their brother for them the best I could.

There were a few times during this meeting that I just wanted to cry my heart out. I felt like I just wanted to fall to my knees and sob. When those feelings came about, I was able to stop talking, close my eyes, and turn around, facing the wall behind me. After a short pause and a prayer, I was able to regain my strength, take a deep breath, turn back around, and make eye contact with them once again and continue on.

It was very difficult to look at each family member and to see the sadness and the concern that they have for Kevin at this time. I saw the tears flowing down their cheeks, along with facial expressions of shock and disbelief. They were confused because nobody in Kevin's family had or has cancer. The doctors told me that this was not hereditary and the siblings should not panic.

Between Lester and me, we were only able to answer some of the questions they had. This was because a lot of the testing still wasn't completed.

After this visit, I decided to go home for a while again. There are still responsibilities that I need to tend to. I needed to be a mom, do laundry, clean the house, and be with the kids. I can always go back to the hospital later on.

When I arrived home, I was surprised to have visitors there already. My brother, Scott; his wife, Brenda; and their kids, Ryan (twenty-six), Jackie (twenty-four), Jessica (eighteen), and Meghan (sixteen), had come over. I've included their ages because I wanted you to realize that on New Year's Eve, I'm sure at this age, they had better things to do than come and help me.

I was excited to see them all. Ryan was home for the holidays from Michigan, where he was transferred for his job, and Jessica was home for college break. Being as Kevin was in the hospital for Christmas, I hadn't had a chance to see them yet. I had arrived home just as they were packing everything up that they had brought with them from home. What a shock and surprise this was for me. I walked into a clean house and saw everything that they had accomplished. I didn't know what to say to any of them.

Once I walked to the kitchen where everyone was, I remember seeing the smiles that they had on their faces. These were smiles of satisfaction that they were able to help us, smiles of "Thank God, we're done," and smiles of love and concern for me. I was stunned at the kindness and support that they had shown us. Evidently they had arrived at 8:00 a.m. in the morning; woke my kids up, which I bet was real fun; and said, "Let's get to work." I bet my kids were surprised!

We had a lot of snow again at this point that needed to be moved. I needed the driveway reopened and snow moved in front of the house. I also needed the snow by our outbuildings and yard cleared so I could get hay in the dry lots for our horses and get to the barn when it needed to be cleaned out.

Scott and Ryan didn't know what we had to work with for snow removal but knew we had some equipment. They brought two different buckets on a trailer from home in hopes that one of them would attach to our tractor or skid loader. Brenda and the kids cleaned the whole house together and did some laundry too. They didn't stop at that either. When they were done with the house, she went to the grocery store and bought food and laundry detergent for the house. It was lunchtime then, so they ordered pizza from the local restaurant and brought it home to have a family meal together.

My heart was empty because Kevin wasn't here to share this time with us, but again I was filled with peace.

Because of Scott and his family, I was able to find the time to go through pictures for a project I wanted to do. I decided that it might be helpful for Kevin if the kids and I put picture boards together and hung them up in his room the next time I went to the hospital. There are many reasons that I thought this would be helpful. When he opens his eyes again, there would be pictures of his family and friends for him to see. It would give his room a more personal feeling and he would see and remember the good times. It may give him some comfort when we aren't there with him to see us in a picture.

I also felt that this would be helpful for the nurses to see the pictures to get to know a little bit more about Kevin. This way, they would have things to talk to him about whenever they were with him.

Kevin's daughter, my stepdaughter, Kaylee, went to see Kevin this afternoon with Nancy, Kevin's sister, and her husband, John. Tony and Stephanie, my children from my previous marriage, weren't ready to see him with all of those tubes yet, so they will visit in a few days.

In the evening, I was very disappointed in the effort the kids put into the picture boards. I really couldn't understand why I had to push them to do this. Didn't they want to help Kevin? Didn't they care? Where did this family time all go?

I know now that they were happy and excited to do this and loved the idea. They just struggled with Kevin being in the hospital, and needing to work together on this project was difficult. Everyone had their own idea of how they wanted it done. Everyone was just tired.

In times of distress and concern, each person reacts differently. There are those who don't want to be reminded that any of this is happening; those who just don't know what to do; some people that you never hear from; those who can't bring themselves to visit; those who want to do it all for you; those who keep close contact with you during an illness; those who know it all; those who pretend that it doesn't bother to them; those who really don't like you, but think that if they show concern and you don't make it, they will feel like they tried; and then those who you know are there for you just because they said they were going to be.

Tonight I called the ICU before I went to sleep, and the nurse said that Kevin was very calm and stable. I said, "Could you please put your . . ." I choked up and couldn't speak, and as I was composing myself, she said, "Yes, Karen, I will put my hand on Kevin and say a prayer for you."

I am so very grateful for all of the support, prayers, and kindness that have been shown to me and my family.

FRIDAY, JANUARY 1, 2010

(update typed SATURDAY, JANUARY 2, 1:41 A.M.)

I hope everyone is feeling well today after last night's festivities. I planned on going to the hospital in the morning to be with Kevin. If the medical staff didn't want me in the room, I would at least be there to check on him from time to time. Before I left home, I called the hospital. I wanted to check on Kevin and confirm an appointment time for the kids and me to meet with the doctors. I feel that it's time for the kids to be involved with a doctor's meeting so they can ask questions.

I was told that Kevin opened his eyes once today already. I was so excited to hear this and wanted to get to the hospital as soon as possible so I too could see his eyes. I was also told that Kevin's blood count is too low today. They don't know why this has happened but have decided to take him for a CT scan. The doctors are concerned that he is losing blood internally from his surgery site.

I hope to have more answers soon and, of course, will keep you updated. A four o'clock appointment had been scheduled for the kids and me to meet with the doctors today. Being as I would already be at the hospital, we needed to decide on a time and place to meet at the hospital. We met in the hospital entrance. I remember seeing them walk down the hall to meet me from the parking garage. I was anxious to lead them to the ICU and show them what was all happening to Kevin. I was feeling so much excitement that we would be together for the first time since December 21. I was also very comforted that they were there with me and Kevin even if it was only for a little while.

Like I said before, everyone reacts differently in these situations. This is the first time that Tony and Stephanie were able or mentally ready to see Kevin. I think they were both nervous and scared of what state they would find Kevin in when they got to the ICU. When we arrived in the ICU, we all went into Kevin's room together at first. It was really nice to see him.

The kids brought the picture boards along that we all had made. We looked around the room and picked the best spot to hang them. We wanted them to be somewhere that he could see right away when he opened his eyes. The nurses came in at this time to greet us and really enjoyed seeing these pictures and listening to the stories we told about each one that we picked. I explained to the kids the reason for each of the tubes that were attached to Kevin. I was hoping that if they knew and saw what their purpose was, they would be more comfortable seeing them.

After a short visit together, I told them that we each should spend some alone time with Kevin before our meeting. I thought that it would be a good idea because there would be no distractions during that time and they could have privacy for their thoughts, words, and feelings.

I know that I said their time with Kevin would be private, but I glanced briefly from outside the room at times. Some would call that nosey, but I felt the need to see how they responded, so I could comfort them.

Kaylee was so scared, but she went first. She wanted her dad to respond to her so badly. I felt bad for her as I watched her search her father's face for something that would make her feel that he was going to be all right. She cried so hard and, at the same time, was trying to understand why this is happening to her dad.

Stephanie was very sad and stunned at the sight of Kevin. I don't think she knew what to do or say to him. I noticed that she held Kevin's hand and talked to him softly but was scared at the same time.

Tony had a hard time even looking at Kevin when we first arrived. I knew he was trying to be strong for us and held back his tears as best as he could. I could see right through him and knew how crushed he was to see Kevin like this. Kevin has always been the man Tony has looked up to for guidance and support.

We were anxious and concerned as to what we would hear at our meeting with the intensive care unit doctor. We met in a private conference room, and I was happy with the one-on-one attention that we received from the medical staff. They explained everything in a brief summary to the kids and made sure all of their questions were answered before continuing on with our meeting.

After the explanation of what had happened to Kevin, we were given the good and bad news. The good news is they found out that Kevin was allergic to a drug called Adavan. This drug was given to him to help with anxiety and his agitation. They had already been giving him this drug for six days. From December 26 through December 31. Whenever Kevin seemed to get more agitated, they increased the dose of this drug. That poor man! I'm disappointed that this happened, but I don't blame the doctors. They were only trying to help him. I am so pleased and relieved that they found this out. Now hopefully we can get on the road to recovery.

Remember that I was told this morning that they needed to find out where he was losing blood. They found no blood loss from the surgical area during the CT scan that was performed earlier today. The doctors are totally stunned. Nobody seems to know where the blood went. I call that nothing but a miracle from God. There is no other explanation. Kevin was taken off the blood thinner due to his low blood count, and they are continuing to watch him closely to try to pinpoint as to why the blood count is going down. Kevin also has developed pneumonia. He is currently being treated with antibiotics in hopes that it will go away.

The bad news is that Kevin unfortunately has Myeloma, which is a type of cancer. Kevin's cancer has already spread into his bone marrow, which is why it is now called Multiple Myeloma. The bone marrow makes the blood cells. Everyone has cancer cells in their body already, but Kevin's cancer cells are trying to take over. Some of these cancer cells had formed into the tumor that attached to his bones and ate away some of his vertebrae.

They still haven't done the bone scan to determine how much cancer there is. This scan will also help to determine if there are other tumors formed already elsewhere in his body. The doctors will do this test as soon as Kevin is fully alert. There is treatment for this cancer but no cure. This means it's possible that the cancer could go into remission for a time. His life could be prolonged in this case and give us an opportunity to be with him longer. We will definitely pray for that.

We are planning that Kevin will start radiation on Monday to kill the tumor on the front side of his neck. Chemotherapy will need to be given to Kevin in the future to kill more cancer cells.

Kevin's breathing is doing well, and they hope to be able to remove the breathing tube tomorrow. If this removal is a success, only 10 to 15 percent of the time will it be necessary for the breathing tube to be put back in due to difficulties.

We have a very strong network of friends and family who are affected by this news and whom we know also feel the pain. It's not easy being positive sometimes, but it really helps in changing my views of this situation.

We are taking the news of cancer *very* hard at the moment. The kids and I have decided that we need to pull together and help each other through this trying time.

When Tony, Kaylee, Stephanie, and I got home, we had a special meeting. During this meeting, we made plans as to what the new rules of the house were going to be. This was a very emotional time for us, but we knew what we needed to do.

Christmas break from school will be ending for the kids, with school resuming on Monday. Life goes on again, and I need to make sure that everyone is going to be all right. I have planned on spending every day that I can at the hospital. I will come home for a while at night to be with the kids and support them in their events. I will then go back to the hospital ICU waiting room at bedtime to be with Kevin for the night. If I can't stay with him in his room, I will stay in the waiting room. In the morning, the kids are more than able to get chores done and get themselves to school, so I will clean up at the hospital and spend the day again.

I asked Tony to be the man of the house during Kevin's absence. I knew this was a huge responsibility for an eighteen-year-old to deal with, but I also knew I could count on him. He was to be responsible for making sure each of them got their homework done, making sure that Stephanie was able to get to her basketball practice and games, and keeping the snow cleared in the yard with the tractor and skid loader.

Kaylee, sixteen years old, was to make sure the house was kept in order, feed the dogs, and help with the meals. She also was to listen to Tony whenever I was not available.

Stephanie was to do all of the horse and cat chores, focus on her studies, and listen to Tony whenever I was not available.

We visited about how sometimes people die instantly and loved ones don't get a chance to tell them that they love them. We still have an opportunity here and are grateful for that. We are blessed to have been together as a family for ten years already, and we are all looking forward to many more. We still have time to become a closer family and make every day the best that we can for each one of us.

Kaylee suggested that we take time and actually do weekly or monthly family nights. We decided that there's no better time to start that but right now. So in the evening, we played some Wii bowling. One of the kids got upset while we were playing the game about something and had decided that she didn't want to do anything with us. She stormed out of the room to be alone. I told her in a stern voice to get back in here, but she replied with a loud "no." The stress of Kevin's illness was evident at this time already for the kids.

At that time, I was exhausted and didn't want any confrontations. I didn't know what to do or say. Tony stepped in and made her come back and sit there to at least be with us, even if she didn't want to play. I was stunned. Wow! Tony! Boy, I guess he already stepped up to the plate for us.

After watching us have some fun for a little while, she decided to join us, and it was very enjoyable.

The evening ended up with another call to the ICU and asking the nurses to pray over Kevin.

We want to, again, thank each and every one of you for your loving thoughts, prayers, and support.

SATURDAY, JANUARY 2, 3:10 P.M.

I have been spending time daily at the hospital. I sit with Kevin in the ICU room as much as the nursing staff allows me to. When I'm not with him, I stand and watch him from outside his room or sit in the waiting room. I try to communicate with the nurses and the doctors as much as possible. It seems like all I do is wait and then wait some more. I wait for Kevin to wake up and for the test results.

Today didn't go as well as we all had planned. This morning, they did a few breathing trials with Kevin, and he did better with them while he was sleeping than he did when he was semi-awake. Kevin had a fever with 101 degrees yet, but the doctors think it was probably due to the infection that he has acquired in his lungs. The doctor's still don't really know what caused the blood loss that had occurred or where it went, but Kevin's hemoglobin blood count is fine today. I know that God was involved with this healing *for sure*!

The goal of the doctors is to get the infection under control first before attempting to take the respirator tube out of Kevin's mouth. I'm hoping that things change for the better as the day progresses and will let you know via e-mail later.

I evidently have had time to think during this time. I've wondered if we were here at this hospital for a special reason. Is there a chance that God has Kevin or me or even both of us here in this circumstance and/or hospital in order to make a difference in something or for someone? I prayed about this and told God that I would try to better understand this trial. I am ready to spread his love, his Word, and testify his miracles to others.

As I was on my way to Kevin's room today, a patient just a couple of rooms down from Kevin's called out to me. She was an elderly woman who thought she knew me. Even though I had no idea who she was, I turned to her with a smile and waved to acknowledge her. A short time later, the nurse had come to me and told me that this woman had been asking for me. She then asked if I would stop by and visit with her for a while to calm her down. I remember going to see this weak elderly woman just one time for a quick greeting and visit, and then I never saw her again. I don't know where she went after our visit.

I have visited and prayed with so many people in the family waiting room. This has given my spirit a lift and has humbled me also. There is always someone or something worse than what you or your loved one is going through.

Other than the two business trips that I have been on, this is the first time in ten years that I haven't seen Kevin or visited with him for such a long period of time. The

37

doctors are concerned with the quantity and quality of rest that I have been getting. Even though I have mastered sleeping in the chairs, the rest I'm getting isn't good enough. They told me that I need to take a break, go home, be with the kids, and just call them anytime I want.

I have children at home that need me too, so I will be going home tonight and staying home tomorrow, Sunday, too. My family, which includes my grandmother, father, mother, sisters and brother, and spouses and their families decided to celebrate Christmas tonight. It will be different without Kevin, but he would want us to go ahead without him. I remember my grandmother, who was ninety-five years old at the time, was very sad for Kevin.

I have commented to some friends about how cold it has been in the house. Both Al and Chris came over to check on this problem and had decided that the molding around three doors needed to be replaced. They felt that too much air is being leaked into the house. We set up a date, and they came and fixed them for me. I still felt cold at home, but it did seem to be better. Maybe it's because I'm tired or something.

I have been asked if I would consider using the Caringbridge website to update everyone on Kevin's condition at all. This would give everyone an opportunity to check on him, not just those who know us personally. I feel that this website is a wonderful way to keep people up to date on a loved one's progress. It's also very inspiring to read the comments and prayers from others, but at the same time, I don't feel that it's confidential. I feel that when a person is writing a comment or prayer on this website, they don't always tell it all because it's not private.

As of now, I would like the replies, the prayers, and the well wishes that are sent our way to be personal and not for everyone to read. I would like those who want to be kept up to date to get added to one of the e-mail lists. I am finding that journaling like this is very therapeutic for me the same as keeping everyone up to date on the news. I have been able to communicate when needed, at any time of day. I have access to a computer at a couple of different areas in the hospital when I don't get journals done at home.

Thank you for the prayers and the support you have shared with us.

There are still *no visitors* or calls allowed yet other than immediate family.

SUNDAY, JANUARY 3

Today was a mix-and-match kind of day. The last thing I do at night before I go to bed is call the ICU nurse, and the first thing I do when I wake up is call the ICU nurse again. This morning started on a more positive note than lately. I was told that when Kevin's eyes had opened during the night, he wasn't really looking at the nurse when he was being talked to but that he was just kind of there. He nodded his head once when asked if he was tired. He was able to squeeze the nurse's hand when asked to during the evening and morning also. They said that Kevin seems to be afraid, which is no surprise to me. He doesn't even know what's happening or where he is.

They will be doing another breathing trial today to see if Kevin can breathe without the respirator yet. Whenever he had done this in the past, he had quite a bit of difficulty when he was semi-alert. He will be monitored again all day.

I felt helpless and concerned but was comforted by going to church. After the church service, a large group of people, the kids, and I gathered at the altar and prayed. We all broke down in tears at times. As I was listening, however, to the prayers being spoken, I felt hope, love, and support. The words that were said were spoken perfectly to represent what we needed.

Later on in the day, Nancy and John were going to see Kevin and be my eyes and hands. I knew they would be very detailed with their visit to me, which was a relief. The doctors asked Nancy to let me know that they want me to come to the hospital tomorrow, Monday, because they are going to try taking the respirator off and feel I should be there for Kevin. The doctors also want to have a family care consult with me in the morning.

We are all in this together for Kevin, and we know that you are praying for his health and well-being also.

MONDAY, JANUARY 4, 1:21 P.M., FIRST E-MAIL

I started the day out being so very excited and prayed that today is the day we can start on the recovery journey together! How do I prepare for this time when it's possible that Kevin will be able to breathe on his own and respond to me? How do I prepare myself to tell the love of my life that he has cancer, and we will be there giving him strength through this? I'm so very excited and hopeful but still am scared at the same time.

I have so many things going through my head that I couldn't sleep last night. I woke up at 3:00 a.m., thinking and wondering if I'd forget anything. Am I going to be prepared? Am I going to be tired? What if I'm tired and don't want to drive home? Will I talk so fast and be excited that Kevin gets overwhelmed again? Will I be able to sleep there? Do the kids come down with me again today? Do I have the necessary phone numbers listed for the kids to call if they need anything?

Today, Tony told me that I shouldn't be driving the green truck until the oil gets changed. How can I do this today? I thought it was really wonderful that Tony paid attention to this detail. The oil level would be okay for just one more day but also knew that I put Tony in charge. I needed to get the oil changed not only because it was due but because Tony was concerned about me.

I was very appreciative of the wonderful local service garage. They knew when I arrived that I was in a hurry and understood the need for me to stay in the vehicle while they changed the oil. I just needed to be alone, relax, and get my head organized. I felt that if I had gotten out, I would have run into someone that would want to talk and I didn't want to at that time. I also thought of the wasted time from walking out of the vehicle to the waiting room and back. I was in a hurry.

While I had alone time in the truck, I was thinking about sending thank you cards to some people who gave us meals, how I needed to shop for supplies for making Kevin a book of the daily updates, the need to clear the snow in the dry lots, etc. I want to make an update book so when Kevin is ready, he can read about what all transpired in this part of his life that he wasn't awake for. It will give Kevin the details that he needs to understand later on. A book would give him the opportunity to read it when he's not so overwhelmed and distraught. Am I too hopeful? Am I setting myself up? Will I be disappointed if Kevin doesn't come out of it today? My mind is racing!

Please keep us all in your prayers today. The kids will be asked many times during the day at school how Kevin is. Please keep them in your prayers also during this time. I will have updates sent to you as soon as I can.

God bless and thank you so very much for your prayers and support.

MONDAY, JANUARY 4, 7:18 P.M., SECOND E-MAIL

I had asked Kevin's brothers, Wally, Lester, and Paul, and sister, Nancy, to meet me at the hospital this morning. I wanted them to be involved in a meeting with the ICU doctors and me because I wanted to be sure there were family members there for additional questions and memory support for myself.

Well, I did it to myself. I got myself so pumped up. I was sure that Kevin was going to need me today. I was hoping that he'd get the respirator off and that the meeting would be informational and be on our way to recovery.

Right now, I'm feeling *really* down. Disappointment doesn't quite cut it. We were all expecting a meeting at 10:00 a.m. for the family care consultation. The doctor was in at 8:00 a.m. and left before we arrived. We were all so disappointed. It wasn't a wasted trip though. We all got to at least see Kevin and touch his hand only for a brief moment.

The radiology that Lester and I were told would happen today wasn't happening either. Actually, now they don't even know when radiology will start. Right now, Kevin has too many tubes attached to him. They would rather do radiology with no tubes. They need to be certain that he doesn't move at all during this process.

All of the siblings that were here this morning had visited Kevin this past weekend. During my visit with them, they told me that they felt that Kevin was doing better today and that every baby step forward is a good thing. One step leads to another and another and so on and so on. I really don't know how they got that he was doing better, but anyway, that's what they said. We just hope that nothing else comes in the way of progress anymore. Before Kevin's family left, they also told me to think of it this way: Kevin was sedated and put on medicine that didn't agree with him for quite a while. It will take some time to heal from it. I know that they are just trying to console me. They don't know what else to say to make me feel better.

Later on, while I was saying good-bye to Kevin, he started getting agitated again. I asked him to squeeze my hand if he needed me to stay. He pressed on my finger and then tried to talk. He opened his eyes, lifted his head, and opened his mouth like he was trying to tell me something. Of course, he couldn't talk; he had a tube in his mouth yet, but he sure tried. His legs started moving all around, and he was getting very agitated again.

The nurse came in suddenly to calm him down. I told her that he wanted me to stay. That he squeezed my finger to stay, but she didn't buy it. Instead I was told that he needs to be alone and rest. She said, "You can call later, but there are no visitors allowed at this time." The nurse also told me that I should call in the morning tomorrow to see if they even want me down here at all.

I felt *terrible*! Do you mean that I couldn't stay by my husband's side like he wanted me to? How in the world do I get him so upset and agitated? Doesn't he know me?

I am totally exhausted, and I promise that I will rest this afternoon. Still no visitors or phone calls please, just keep praying.

I received this e-mail from my friend Theresa and thought that it would be very appropriate to share with you.

> Karen, you mentioned that what is happening to all of you does make a difference in **all** of our lives . . . you are right.
>
> It makes us not take our health for granted and our loved ones for granted. It makes it so we don't feel so sorry for ourselves over the trivial matters in life when we know someone we care about is going through the most difficult things imaginable.
>
> I am reminded of a scripture verse that helped me a lot in the last two years. I know that God gave it to me and I found it in many places when I did not even expect it.
>
> "Wait on the Lord. Be of good courage and He will strengthen your heart."
>
> God did not say He was necessarily going to take away the problem, but that He will give my heart what it needs to endure.
>
> God bless you!
>
> Love,
> Theresa

TUESDAY, JANUARY 5
(update typed THURSDAY, JANUARY 7, 1:51 A.M.)

I didn't e-mail yesterday because I had a *really* bad day. As the day went on, I did get stronger but got let down again at night when I called the ICU. I was told that they noticed from a scan performed earlier in the day that Kevin's liver showed signs of damage. I also was told that they had questions about his brain scan and more testing would need to be done. I was so concerned and didn't know how to take this news.

I went to Tony's basketball game at the high school in the evening. I just love to watch our kids play basketball, and I needed to support him too. During warm-ups, I love counting how many three-point baskets Tony makes in a row. When he misses, I just start counting over. It seems I can't get enough of this. Not only did I get to watch Tony play, but I got to watch our girls play their instruments in the pep band. I also felt that we needed to let the community know and see that we are okay and that it's all right to talk about Kevin. There are many who are concerned and need personal interaction.

Tony, however, is having a hard time with this right now. He has told me that *everyone* is asking him about Kevin. He is sick of repeating everything to everyone, so he resided to telling them either "Kevin's fine" or "I don't know." This way, the subject is dropped or changed. The fact that he felt like this really bothered me, but I didn't push the issue.

I thought that Tony didn't care about us and that he didn't even want to know what was going on. I realize now that I was so very wrong. I was thinking of others in getting the information told and not of my son's feelings. Tony just needed a break from talking and explaining this topic.

It's like a mountain that just gets plopped down in front of you, knowing that you need to climb it, being frustrated and scared, and needing help from others to make it. Sometimes you just want to quit and pretend that the mountain is not there. I feel that's where Tony was. He wanted to have times that he didn't need to think of us and Kevin's cancer. In the end, we will make it to the top of this mountain. I am sure we will come across cliffs and stumbling rocks along the way. Our faith, support, and love from friends and family will pick us up and keep us strong all of the way.

WEDNESDAY, JANUARY 6
(update also typed THURSDAY, JANUARY 7, 1:51 A.M.)

Kevin did look better today. His tongue, wrists, and ankles were not as swollen as they had been.

Today, Nancy and I drove together to Abbott for a consultation with the ICU doctors. This was a lot of information to take in, but this is what we got.

The bad news is that the doctors want to wait at least four more weeks or so to do the radiation treatment on the remaining tumor. This is because the surgeon that rebuilt his neck wants the bone graft in his C2 vertebra to take hold or heal better first. Kevin currently has cancer in 30 to 40 percent of his bone marrow. Protein studies show his cancer is in stage 2. He needs a stem cell transplant in order to prolong his life.

My concern at this time was wondering if the delayed radiation treatment would give time for the cancer to spread. There is nothing that I know of that could change that other than prayers.

The stem cell transplant includes harvest or collection of his cells once they are in remission. Kevin will need to take medication to kill cancer cells in order to get into remission. He will then need chemotherapy to wipe out his bone marrow of cells as best as it can. When the chemotherapy is done, they will then transplant his own stem cells that were previously cleaned and collected back in his system to prolong his life.

The doctors are currently giving Kevin a drug intravenously, used for delirium. An antipsychotic drug called Saraquill. When Kevin is ready for chemotherapy, it will be given to him in the form of a pill.

Kevin has a fever again today, ranging from 101 to 102 degrees. We were told that the high fever doesn't always necessarily mean it's from pneumonia. They really don't have an answer for this at this time.

His agitation could be due to a number of reasons: postoperative pain, the tube in the throat, and the respirator in his mouth.

The medical staff thinks that it's possible that Kevin would do better without the respirator in his mouth. If they remove the respirator, it would need to be replaced with a tracheotomy. The doctors don't even want to talk about a tracheotomy for at least three to four more days. They want to give Kevin some more time but will do one if there is no other choice. One of the reasons for not doing the tracheotomy is that they don't know if he will tolerate the removal of the respirator due to his uncontrollable agitation and breathing.

Kevin's secretions are getting thicker and most of them have checked positive for strep throat. The secretions could be caused from the respirator tube due to the long length of time it has been in his throat. Kevin's ammonia, triglyceride levels and blood pressure are very high. They feel it is due to the side effects of the drugs Kevin has been and is currently taking. The doctors feel these levels will go down as he is weaned off the medications. The propofol medication that was being administered was making the fat go up in Kevin's blood. They are taking him completely off of that drug.

Good news is that Kevin's kidney functions and calcium levels are okay. I was also informed that the bad news I received last night in regard to his liver and brain was false information. His liver seems to be in good working order today, and he didn't have a brain scan before today, so there was nothing to report on yesterday in regard to this. I was confused with the liver information but thought this was good news and really didn't care about how this happened.

When Nancy and I left the hospital today, they were taking Kevin for some MRIs: one on his head to check his brain, one on his neck to check on his operative area, and one on his chest.

What do I say? Who would have thought it would have been Kevin?

Our friend, Dean, called me and asked if I needed any snow moved yet. What a relief! I really didn't have time to figure out who I'd ask to do this for me or when I would have time to do it myself. There was so much snow in the dry lots due to the snowstorm. When Scott and Ryan were here plowing snow, they didn't even think of doing these. Whenever the snow slides off the roof in the dry lot, the passage for the animals to the shelter is very difficult, and that's where I have their hay. It also needed to be done because when the piles of snow start to melt, they will refreeze into ice as soon as it gets colder again. This would make snow removal very difficult in the spring and cause flooding of the lean two's besides. The lean two's are overhang shelters for the animals and where I put the hay.

Dean was glad to help and told me when he would be able to come over so I could show him what I needed done.

Later on in the day, I went back to spend some time at the hospital again. It was youth group night at church, and the kids won't be home anyway for me to spend time with until later on.

I'm grateful for all of the help, food, and support we have received from everyone. We are so very blessed to have each one of you sending your thoughtfulness and prayers. We will continue to need them, as this will be a long journey, and we know we won't be alone.

Thursday, January 7, 2:16 p.m., first e-mail

I called the hospital early this morning, and the report I was given seems to be better news so far.

Kevin is weaning well off of the drugs, he is CPAP-ing well. CPAP-ing is breathing with the help of the ventilator support. "With the help of the ventilator" means that he is breathing a little bit on his own too. How wonderful! We are all praying that Kevin will continue the good work and be able to get the respirator off today. He is less sedated and not as restless or agitated as he had been in the past.

Kevin, however, does have pneumonia and *a lot* of secretions. The medical staff is trying to remove as much of them as possible with a suction tube. This is very uncomfortable for Kevin.

I don't know yet if the nurses want me at the hospital or not today. I sure hope they say yes. When I called again midmorning, the nurse told me that our minister and six or so others came in earlier. They stood around Kevin's bed and prayed with him. What a wonderful blessing this was for us! Pastor Joel told me later on that Kevin knew they were there. He told me that it looked as if Kevin was trying to tell them thank you!

It's so very hard for me not being there with him.

I have been trying to keep Kevin's checkbook and our bills up to date. Kevin had handled the family checkbook, and I had handled the farm account checkbook. I'm used to balancing each monthly bank statement, and he's not. I wasn't aware of which bills had automatic payment schedules and which were not. I didn't realize how fast the money was being spent because I haven't looked at these bills for a long time. I didn't know the passwords for accounts and didn't know where he kept them either. I took it for granted that Kevin would always take care of this. He hasn't been awake or able to answer any questions I had, so I figured it out on my own.

I started my own filing system and did my best on reconciling the checkbook. When a check would be written, Kevin always rounded up the dollar amount in the checkbook register, so it showed he had less money than he really does. This makes it impossible to reconcile the check book.

THURSDAY, JANUARY 7, 11:57 P.M., SECOND E-MAIL

It ended up that I was able to be with Kevin in the early afternoon. Due to Kevin's agitation, the doctors decided to try to remove the respirator. They sedated him *a lot* before they did the procedure in order to make sure that his airway was open enough. At two thirty, it was a success. The respirator had been removed. I bet that feels so much better for him. We've been praying for this for what seems to be quite a while now. Thank you, God, once again!

The nurse told me at 4:00 p.m. that all of Kevin's vitals are good for now, but he still gets anxious. When he gets anxious, they will adjust his meds just a little bit to calm him back down.

Kevin has been very confused at times today. He thinks it is December right now and that Christmas is coming soon. He also at times thinks he is in the gym with the therapist or in the doctor's office. When I thought about this, he really did miss all of this time. What a blessing it is that he doesn't remember any of what had gone on this whole time. I guess they gave him drugs to forget. We will celebrate Christmas with him when he gets home from the hospital.

Kevin currently is given oxygen by use of a humidity mask because of his sore throat. He can't talk yet but can whisper just a little.

I went home so Kevin could get some much-needed rest. Tomorrow is another day.

What a difference from yesterday! God heard all of our prayers last night and even this morning at 4:00 a.m., when I was pleading with him to calm Kevin so the doctors could help him.

Tomorrow I will call the doctor's office after 10:00 a.m. to see if Kevin is up to any visitors. I told the nurse that I wouldn't talk too much or get too excited this time in hopes to stay in the room with him. She didn't even laugh at that statement this time.

We still have a *long* way to go with this illness with good and bad days ahead. I know we won't be alone in this journey. God is an awesome God who heals. I know he has heard our prayers and has brought Kevin this far in the healing process.

Thank you for all of the support and prayers you have given us. I think I know some people who will sleep better tonight.

FRIDAY, JANUARY 8, 10:29 P.M.

I called this morning around 10:00 a.m. to see if I could come to the hospital to see Kevin. The nurse told me that the respirator *and* the feeding tube were removed, but Kevin is not cooperating with them at all. She told me that Kevin keeps trying to stand up and says he's going home. He is very determined to leave. They let me talk to him on the phone in hopes that I could calm him down. It worked! I was able to make him understand. I told him that he still was very sick and convinced him to stay put at the hospital. I said that I would come right away to be with him and asked if he needed me to bring him anything from home. He told me to bring a shotgun. The stories he said to me at this time were great!

It was so wonderful to hear his voice even if he wasn't able to speak other than a whisper. He didn't make sense of what he was trying to tell me at times. I can imagine how confused he must be right now.

I made it to the hospital as fast as I could. When I arrived in his ICU room, the nurse asked him who I was. Kevin said, "That's my wife." Then he said, "I love her." What wonderful words to hear from him. I was so happy I didn't even need to ask him if he loved me this time. He just said it.

While Kevin and I were visiting, some of what he said wasn't making sense to me at all, but I didn't care. He was awake, his eyes were opened, and the tube was out of his mouth.

Kevin had been strapped to the bed for twelve days now. Because of this, he was in need of therapy. His strength went away very fast. His hands were so weak, and he needed help even holding utensils to feed himself with.

The physical therapist came to work with him today for the first time. There was one set of exercises for the hands that was difficult for him to do. It was even hard for me to understand how to do what she had asked of him. I saw that he was having a difficult time so I tried to move his hand to help him. Oh my! With a quick jerk of his hand and piercing eyes glaring at me, I knew that he wanted to do it himself. I was proud of his determination and understood his need to succeed.

The lunch tray came, and Kevin wanted to eat right away. I didn't know if he was that hungry or determined to feed himself. The tray was placed in front of him, and I noticed that he was trying to scoop the food onto the spoon. Seeing how much of a struggle this was for him, I asked if I could help him. I made sure that I asked first this time. He said "yes." I put food on the spoon for him and assisted just a little to get his hand to his mouth.

When the nurse came in, I had told her what he accomplished. She told me in a stern voice that under no circumstance was I to let him do that. The amounts of food on each spoon needed to be limited. This was to be sure that he was able to swallow it all really good before the next spoonful. I didn't do any of that! We got in trouble the first day already. I must have been out of the room when they gave him instructions to wait for the nurse or the therapist to come and feed him. He was so determined to feed himself that he wouldn't wait.

He had then asked for our friend, Al, to come and see him. I cleared it with the nurses, and when Al arrived a short while later, the shit was flying. They were teasing and telling stories one after another. It was so much fun! Some of what Kevin was saying made sense and some didn't. Out of the blue, he became angry. He started telling Al a story of what he thought had happened. He said, "She totaled out our truck! She ran it into the side of the hospital!" Boy was he mad. I consoled him and told him that it didn't happen and it must have been a dream. He, of course, didn't believe me.

We'd be talking and all of a sudden, Kevin would laugh. We'd ask him what was funny, and he'd start saying something and make sound effects. This went on for a while, and we made the visit short. When Kevin got tired, he didn't hesitate to tell us to leave.

What a wonderful day! I loved to see him smile and laugh again!

You know when I said that Kevin was whispering lightly, smiling, and laughing quite a bit? Well, in the later afternoon, he became frustrated, confused, restless, and nonstop again. I was concerned and wondering if we were going backward again. I was disappointed and sad that what I saw earlier in the day was gone.

I'm going to stay at the hospital overnight to check on him from time to time. I don't want to go all of the way home and then find out that he needed me during the night. Kevin is still not accepting visitors other than family, and even that is limited for right now.

Hopefully, Kevin will be starting more physical therapy on Monday and be back on the floor in his own room soon. I can only imagine how much more comfortable it would be for both of us.

SATURDAY, JANUARY 9, 5:56 P.M., FIRST E-MAIL

While yesterday, Friday, was a good day and a positive step forward for Kevin, he still had a very restless night. He was still feeling the effects of the drugs and was confused and agitated at times. Put it this way, we didn't get much sleep again last night at all! I got one hour, and I don't really know if he got any. His body was moving the whole time, and he was trying to get out of bed. It was constant!

Every once in awhile, Kevin thought there were mice crawling on his legs and biting him. We think it's because of the braces that he needs to wear on his legs. The braces get pumped up with air and release it again to keep the blood circulating in his legs. This probably feels like mice crawling or something. He kept kicking his legs and getting very agitated. He would yell that there are rats in the rafters. He'd say, "Shh, can't you hear them? They are all over!" Then, it was quiet and all of a sudden, he would look out into the hallway and think he saw an old classmate of his.

Kevin was telling me that he missed the Super Bowl, and he was really mad. When I told him that it's January and the Super Bowl wasn't played yet, he argued with me. He also kept getting mad because he was still saying that someone took our truck and ran it into the hospital and wrecked it. I think this is why he asked me to bring the shotgun from home. Kevin had asked me to sleep in bed with him, but I said, "There are too many cords, and I can't. I'll need to stay in the recliner next to you instead for tonight." As long as I was going to stay in the room with him, he was all right with that.

Throughout the night, he kept trying to get out of bed again. Whenever I couldn't control him, I called for a nurse to help me. For the most part, the nursing staff was excellent and easy to deal with. I only had one instance that was unacceptable and pissed me off.

Kevin's regular ICU nurse went on break around 3:00 a.m. She had told me who was covering for her in case I needed help.

Well, Kevin was uncontrollable around 3:10 a.m., and I called for the covering nurse to help me. She came in that room and was so mad at me. She actually told me, "This is a privilege that you can even be here in the room with your husband. If you can't control him, I'm going to have you leave the room."

As soon as we got him stable, I asked if I could stay, and she said, "Not in here, only in the waiting room."

I couldn't believe this! I tried to rest but kept thinking of Kevin. I checked on him thirty minutes later to find that he was *out of bed and standing alone*. No nurse was even close! That did it! I yelled for her, and she came running. She didn't say a word when I took over in the room or when I pulled up my recliner next to his bedside for me to stay and sleep on for that matter either. I actually never had that nurse as a backup or anything again after that.

The regular nurse came back on duty, and we were not able to calm him down until midmorning. The nurses wanted him to rest more today and have requested that he not have any visitors at this time. He is alert enough to know that I am there for him at the hospital, so I am staying to help keep an eye on him.

Kevin received the following e-mail which was helpful for me to read today.

> DON'T ask God why me, DON'T blame God and DON'T make promises to God that you can't or won't keep. THANK him daily for the breathe you are able to breathe, for the sight to see your families faces, to feel their hand on yours, for the sun that warms you up and the rain that nourishes the earth, for the friends that make you smile and another day of life.
>
> Pray each day as a new day and not as the previous day or the next day to come because what's happen is the past is unchangeable and the future is what God allows and what we make it to be.
>
> Use the energy from your frustration and anger in positive ways, as hard as it may be at times. DO NOT ALLOW this energy to wear you down the cancer can do that on its own. It does not need your help.
>
> Be excited for even the small things you accomplish, don't weigh yourself down with the things you cannot do right now because one day, you will be able to again remember. It's the small things that keep us trying to do more.
>
> We love you very much!

SATURDAY, JANUARY 9, SECOND E-MAIL

Saturday, midday, the nurse took blood samples and did Kevin's vitals. The ICU doctor also visited with Kevin and me, explaining that they had been weaning Kevin off of the medicines that kept him from hallucinating gradually for the last day or two. Yesterday he was totally taken off of them. This is probably why he had such a difficult time in the afternoon and evening hours. The nurse was told to go ahead and re-administer small doses of this medication again to Kevin only periodically to help as needed. She also reassured me that Kevin will heal just fine from this setback of drug reactions. Sometimes it just will take a little bit longer to recover.

Later on, I didn't know what to do with myself when Kevin was settled and comfortable. I really wasn't needed there at the time. I felt I had things that I needed to do at home. I needed to check on the kids and thought they would appreciate a break from chores. I didn't know if I should go home, stay here in the family waiting room and do some paperwork, give Kevin time alone, or stay by his side. I had a very difficult time leaving Kevin, but I had decided to go home and see what happens. I can always come back. I'm getting used to the drive by now.

When I arrived home, I did some things around the house and found out that the kids were busy and had made plans. Nobody was going to be home for the evening. I guess it didn't pay for me to stay home alone. I called the hospital to double-check that I could come back and stay in Kevin's room with him again. Because Kevin has been such a handful and uncontrollable most of the time, the medical staff asked me if I would stay through the night and the morning. They told me that if I couldn't, they would have had to hire a babysitter to stay in his room with him. I thought Kevin would be more comfortable with me than a stranger but wanted the staff to ask him to see what he wanted.

The nurse came back on the phone with Kevin's answer being, "Sure! Tell her to bring her homemade salsa for the nurses and some food for me too!" He doesn't like the hospital food at all. Because of all that had happened and the possible difficulty in swallowing, he has to have a special diet for a few days. This diet consists of pureed food, and it tastes terrible.

I was able to find a few food items that would work with his diet for a day or so. I packed up the food, got cleaned up, finished chores, and got my bag ready for the night at the hospital. I was so excited that he chose for me to come instead of a babysitter. I really wanted it that way.

Well, tonight, Kevin was pretty good so far. It is just so nice to be able to visit with him. We have so much to talk about. He has already been able to speak stronger today than yesterday. We both are really tired, and I am really looking forward to a calm night tonight. We are anticipating and hoping that Kevin will get moved to a room tomorrow on the eighth floor and will be allowed visitors soon.

Each day, we have been blessed with prayers, kindness, and help from friends, family, and the community. Words can't even start to explain how much we appreciate all of the support we've received.

SUNDAY, JANUARY 10, 4:49 P.M.

Last night, Saturday, was a much better night. Kevin had difficulty only two or three times during the night. The third time, he wasn't listening to me anymore and was trying to get out of bed by himself again. After the nurses tucked him back in bed, he still was very agitated.

Kevin looked at me and said, "Get in," and patted the bed with his hand. After Friday night's fiasco, I found room this time and got onto the bed. It felt so wonderful to feel his arm around my waist even if it was for only thirty minutes. He rested his head on mine, which was kind of heavy, but so what, and then he fell asleep. Once I felt he was sleeping hard enough, I quietly and gently slid off the bed to return to my recliner. I was concerned that I would accidentally mess up the tubes.

It was a record. He slept from 3:20 a.m. until 7:10 a.m. He seemed confused again this morning at first but as he woke up more, we were talking about the Olympics, etc. He did much better. His sense of humor was back too. He told me that when his catheter gets taken out, he will have to be potty trained again. He thought that was pretty funny. It was so nice to see and hear him laugh and smile again.

There are four times per day that nobody is able to be in the ICU area or even in the patient's room in the ICU. This is downtime for the patients and for the nurses to do their records. Being as Kevin and I are working so well together again today, the staff had asked me to stay during this ICU downtime to keep an eye on him. They feel that this will be a tremendous help to the nursing staff. This way they can get what they need done and not always need to be with Kevin to settle him down.

I hope our kids come and visit Kevin soon. I know how happy that would make him. Kaylee will stop in after her softball practice today. She is going to wear her uniform to the hospital to surprise Kevin. He has been asking about all of the kids' sporting events, knowing that he's missed some games.

Kevin is talking stronger each day and has really been determined whenever he does his exercises. He stood three times yesterday, while transferring from the bed to the chair and has already done it once again this morning.

Kevin told me this morning, "I really don't like that nurse who feeds me. She always pushes her food on me. It tastes like shit and wants me to eat it anyway. She does this just so she can walk away with the profits from the food."

Hope to have a great day, and please keep the prayers coming.

Chapter 4

RECOVERY AND SET BACKS

Unbelievably the medical staff felt things were going in the right direction. We were transferred out of the ICU and back to the eighth floor of the hospital later on in the evening. It seemed like eternity for the paperwork to clear to switch departments. I had everything from the room together for the move and was anxiously waiting along with Kevin.

As long as things were going better and we were on our way out of the ICU, I felt it was time to inform Kevin about his cancer. How do I even start to explain this to him? I rehearsed the words to myself over and over again and have thought about how hard it would be to tell him and tried to plan how I would do this. I sat by his side and held his hand with tears swelling in my eyes and said that I had something to talk to him about. Kevin instantly looked at me and said "I'm so relieved to get out of the ICU and on the way to recovery. No news is good news and I must not have cancer." Wow, this will be such a let down and shock to him. I mean we all knew about this for what seems to be such a long time already and have somewhat got over the shock and learned to deal with it. Instantly the words came out of my mouth. I said "The test results showed that the tumor is cancerous and that the cancer is in your bone marrow." I mean, wow! I said it! He said, "I guess I was wrong." This was very devastating for Kevin.

Currently he has been in a state of confusion, drug reaction, hallucinating, and restlessness since December 26. He had no idea about any of this and now I hit him with this news! The quiet moment that followed, along with some tears from both of us, seemed to last forever. We just hugged and prayed while having a sincere, private moment between the love of my life, whom I'd do anything for, and me.

It is so scary to be going to the unknown with this disease or anything for that matter. Nobody could have prepared us for the journey that lies ahead of us. We know that we aren't the only family to have this challenge and unfortunately won't be the last

51

family either. Even though the illnesses may be the same, there probably still wouldn't be the same story and outcome for any families.

After a short while, we were informed that the move was secured. The reason it took so long for our transfer is that the eighth-floor nurses were hesitant in getting Kevin back in their care. I don't know how they did it, but we were transferred that night. I feel that it was too late in the evening to transfer because it would be a new situation and it would be hard to get settled and relax.

Monday, January 11, first e-mail

Last night, Kevin didn't sleep at all. We were in totally different surroundings, with unfamiliar nurses. I'm sure he was upset with so many different thoughts going through his mind. He was just told the news of being diagnosed with cancer.

Once, when I woke up, I checked on Kevin. His eyes were wide open, and he looked like he couldn't move. I went over to him and asked if he was okay. He said, "Every time I move in bed, it makes a sound. It's too loud, and I can't sleep with that all night long." Being as he is well known on this floor, he also got tethered to an alarm. If he moves too much or tries to get out of bed without a nurse present or any help, an alarm goes off.

Monday, January 11, second e-mail

This morning, Dr. Schwartz came to see Kevin. While standing by his bedside, he said, "Good morning, Mr. Erickson. My name is Dr. Schwartz. I have been working on your case since you've arrived here at Abbott. The tests results came back and you have a cancer called Multiple Myeloma." Wow! What terrible bedside manner this doctor had! I couldn't believe it. He didn't even know if I had talked to him yet or not. He just blurted it out! No preparation, no explanation, no nothing. Just a "you have a cancer called Multiple Myeloma."

Thank you, God, for giving me the insight for telling Kevin last night about the cancer. The timing was just right. He was at least prepared for this but still was shocked at how this doctor told him. After the short visit with the doctor, Kevin went for the bone survey. This survey will determine if there are any more tumors attached to any other bones. Kevin told me that they took at least sixty-five x-rays, and it took a full hour to complete. The results from the bone survey will be discussed at tomorrow's meeting with Kevin's siblings, Kevin, and me.

Today was the first day Kevin was fully alert, with no strays of his mind. He had been in the ICU since December 28. That's fifteen days! Do you believe it? He is an amazing and determined man for sure. The nurses, both in the ICU and on the eighth floor, commented that they have been watching his progress. They all said that it is a *miracle* as to how well he is doing.

Kevin was assisted in walking with the walker for a while today already. His vitals are great, and his temperature is still down and good.

My sister, Penny, and her husband visited tonight. This was very emotional for all of us. We appreciated them stopping by once again, and it was really nice to see them. After they had left, I went to get some of the get-well cards that had been sent to Kevin. I pulled up a chair along his bedside and asked him if he was up to reading them with me. Kevin and I, then, sat together and read the cards and visited for about forty-five minutes. I asked him if he wanted to quit and read them at a later date, but he said, "No. Keep reading." I'm not sure what this made him feel like other than probably sad and encouraged at the same time.

Hopefully, tonight, Kevin sleeps well. Tomorrow at 8:15 a.m. is our meeting with the doctors, and we both really need our rest so we're alert.

Tuesday, January 12

The doctor reviewed the details of the cancer illness that Kevin has at our morning meeting. The details are that the Multiple Myeloma has infected 35 to 40 percent of his bone marrow at this time. The bone survey that was taken this past Monday showed that there are no other bones in Kevin's body with a cancerous tumor on them. This is wonderful news! The tumors are centralized to the upper spine. Part of the tumor was already removed, and the other part that's attached to the front of his vertebrae is still there. Kevin will not need another surgery to remove it because they will try to remove it with radiation treatment.

Dr. Schwartz is going to a conference tonight at the Mayo Clinic and will discuss Kevin's case with a doctor who specializes in this cancer. He feels that this doctor would be a good doctor to have on our medical team because they are currently having great success in a new medication in treating it. He could give us insight as to what is the best thing for us to do.

So far we have choices. We can do physical therapy to get him strong and walking here at first and then he can be transferred to outpatient therapy back home. We can also start radiation either at Abbott or Waconia and do chemo and bone marrow transplant down the road at the Mayo *or* do therapy here at Abbott and everything else down at the Mayo Clinic in Rochester. This would include radiation, chemo, and the transplant.

We discussed this and decided that we would like Kevin to get therapy at the Sister Kenny Institute. This institute is well known for success and is attached to the Abbott Hospital here. In order to get in for therapy, you need to be approved. Before Kevin can even move or start therapy, he needs to have an assimilation done. Assimilation is a test that will determine what parts of the body needs radiation. We also decided that the Mayo Clinic is exactly where we would want to go for the chemotherapy and stem cell transplant. It is wonderful that our doctor will work with us to get us there.

After the meeting, Kevin's siblings left and we had some alone time to regroup and analyze our decisions.

We were both just relaxing, feeling like the crazy reactions to the medications are now done. We have a plan and now realize some of the things that are ahead of us at least.

Later on, Kevin was on the computer *and* doing things *he wasn't supposed to do*. He was standing on his own, without a helper. Can you believe that he was standing and walking two to four steps from the chair to the bench with nothing to hang on to? After all this?! He is a very determined man, which is good because he will fight this disease with the help of God, but he isn't thinking at all of what could happen if he would fall.

Well, he didn't listen to me all morning when I repeatedly had asked him to ask for help from the nurses or me when he wanted to move. I was really frustrated with this because he was putting himself in danger again. Mind you, as far as the hospital was concerned, he still needed a babysitter with him at all times. Well, I had enough. I left because he wasn't listening to me. I turned him into the nurses, telling them what he was doing. I was hoping that they could set him straight. I needed to go home anyway because I had errands that I needed to do, and in the early evening, Stephanie had a basketball game that I needed to attend.

Our kitchen sink had been leaking for some time now. Lately it has gotten much worse. It was leaking so bad that it was spraying on the floor at this time. I mentioned this to our friend, John, and he offered to fix it for me. He's even coming over as soon as tomorrow to fix it so I need to buy a new one for a replacement today.

While I was gone, some staff from the Sister Kenny Institute met with Kevin and tested him on a few things. They needed to see if he would qualify for their program and might be able to notify us as soon as tomorrow as to if Kevin was accepted or not. I had an enjoyable night out and about with friends at the game and was able to go back again to the hospital to be with Kevin.

He must have gotten caught getting out of bed and doing stuff that he wasn't supposed to do. I guess a certain nurse really chewed him out royally while I was gone. When I came back to the hospital after Steph's game, Kevin said "That one nurse was so mad at me. She was pointing her finger at me and everything!" He said that every time he wanted to move to a chair or do anything after that, he made sure that he called the nurse for assistance.

We actually managed to relax at 10:00 p.m. and watched a Clint Eastwood movie together. I even got to snuggle with Kevin for a while during this time because he was finally tube-free. What freedom this must be for him to not have any tubes connected to him anymore. We always needed to be so very careful around them. As soon as he fell asleep and I knew he was content, I went to my couch for some needed rest.

Sometimes, we need to be reminded of the events that have happened to realize the miracles that go on daily. I praise God for answering our prayers, and I thank you for partnering together for Kevin.

Kevin can finally accept visitors at this time.

Pastor Joel came to see us, and his message was from Philippians 4, starting at verse 4: "Don't worry, trust in the Lord and peace will guard our hearts and minds."

When we worry, we are leaving room for the Devil to work his way in, unless we trust in the Lord completely. Give praise for the miracles he has already shown us.

I just want to let you know of some of the miracles that have happened, showing proof that God has been carrying Kevin throughout this time. Now you know that Kevin was bedridden for twenty-one days. During this whole time, Kevin had been struggling and straining all of his muscles *a lot*! I mean he would pull with his hands and feet and try to sit up. Ever since Kevin has been able to communicate with us, he *has never had pain* or *stiff muscles*. He didn't reinjure his neck, where he had surgery, even while pushing off his tight brace or lifting his head with little support. Not only that but when you think about it, Kevin's feet never left the bed, other than him trying to escape all of the time. He still didn't go anywhere.

Well, Monday morning, Kevin stood a few times throughout the morning and early afternoon. Later in the afternoon, the physical therapist walked with Kevin for a hundred feet with the walker and did eight steps. Everyone was impressed with this miraculous progress also. Sunday night was also the first night that I felt that his hallucinations might have been gone for good.

WEDNESDAY JANUARY 13, 7:38 P.M.

Dr. Schwartz came to visit with us early in the morning. He told us that he had talked to Dr. Kumar from the Mayo Clinic sometime yesterday about Kevin's case. After some review of the situation, Dr. Kumar said that he wants Kevin to do his fifteen or so radiation treatments here at the Sister Kenny Institute. Then he wants to see Kevin at the Mayo Clinic for an evaluation on his progress within four to six weeks from now. Kevin could be eligible to participate in a study before any chemotherapy or bone marrow transplant is discussed.

If Kevin is accepted and completes physical therapy at Sister Kenny before completion of the radiation, I will drive him back to Abbott for the remaining treatments on a daily basis. Kevin and I do feel very positive about what has been decided.

Marilyn from the Sister Kenny Institute visited us this morning around 9:30 a.m. She told us that Kevin had been accepted to receive the beginning physical therapy there. How wonderful that is for us. We won't know how long this therapy will take until after Kevin had a couple sessions. At that time, the doctor's will have to reevaluate Kevin closer to see how well he handles normal activities. If more therapy is needed after Kevin's stay here at Abbott, he will transfer to Howard Lake Rehab for outpatient therapy.

She asked many questions about our living conditions for Kevin in order to determine if we could accommodate his handicap at home. She was satisfied with the fact that I would be able to be with him at all times because he still is in need of 24/7 care and supervision. It is also very helpful that he is able to be on one level at home for everything. She did inform me of the necessary things that would need to be done in order for Kevin to come home. Things like bath rails, shower rails, railing for the two steps to Kevin's living room, a bath chair, a wheelchair, a walker, and a cane.

I called my brother-in-law, John, and visited with him about what the institute told us. I was able to meet with him at Menards after lunch to purchase the necessary items that would work for us.

John is so talented at this kind of thing, and he reassured me that he would take care of putting it all together for us. I felt comforted that it would be done in time for us to come home and it would be done the right way.

After shopping, I returned home to meet with our friend, John. He came over to replace our sink. I felt so bad for him. Our old sink was so corroded and on so tight that it was so very hard for him to get the old sink off. He did manage to finish replacing it, and I was so grateful.

The kids had religion that night, so I was able to go back to the hospital earlier than normal.

A friend wrote the following in a card that they sent to us: "Without faith, nothing is possible, but with it nothing is impossible."

Thank you for your continued support and prayers.

Thursday, January 14, 1:08 p.m.

Yesterday, we were told that Kevin would undergo radiation at the same time as being at the Sister Kenny Institute, but there has been a change. The radiation has been postponed again. Is this a bad thing? Is the cancer growing as we speak because it isn't being treated? The surgeon's didn't want radiation until four weeks or so after surgery because they want the bone graft on his vertebrae to heal better.

Kevin will be moving to the institute today.

Chris and Judy popped in before the move for a short visit, and they were so amazed at how well Kevin looked and was doing. It was so nice to see them again. Kevin and Chris coached baseball and basketball together for years and have become good friends. Judy is a nurse, so I felt good about her comment on how good Kevin looked. I knew I could trust her honesty too. See, this has been a miracle!

Please keep Kevin in your prayers for the rest, the strength, the comfort, and the healing he needs.

This next step is going to be a challenge for Kevin because he's not used to being weak and needing help from others. After Kevin had moved to the institute, we met with a nurse. She gave us a tour and informed us of what goes on in the institute. It's a whole new ball game here. It's very structured, monitored, and busy. Kevin will get a schedule the night before to let him know his therapy schedule for the next day. He will do a total of three hours of therapy but will be broken up in segments.

For example, tomorrow 8:00 a.m. to 9:00 a.m., occupational therapy; 11:00 a.m. to 11:30 a.m., speech therapy; 11:30 a.m. to noon, physical therapy; 1:00 p.m. to 1:30 p.m., occupational therapy; 2:00 p.m. to 2:30 p.m., physical therapy; 2:30 p.m. to 3:00 p.m., another physical therapy. His days are pretty full, so I will be going home during the day to get things done and come back to visit after his appointments are done.

Kevin really isn't up to phone calls or many visitors anyway at this time. He is going to be a tired man by the end of the day, and I don't expect to be able to be with him for very long at each visit.

Kevin will need to be able to dress himself at therapy before they would even consider releasing him. Just the thought of the possibility of not being released was terrifying to him, I'm sure. Kevin told me before I left that he needs some bigger clothes. The shirts he has with him now aren't big enough to go over his neck brace. Bigger clothes would make it so much easier for him to get himself dressed. We are praying that Kevin can pass the therapy tests pretty soon so he can come home and continue therapy locally and be with all of us.

I am so blessed that you all were right there for Kevin and me in this chapter of our lives. When you think about it, Kevin just found out he had cancer, unlike us who have been dealing with this since December 24. We had a number of weeks to wonder, cry, hope, and question the situation. Kevin was given the facts and all of them for that fact in just five days. I think he needs time to think, cry, and pray.

Please also pray for me for rest, organization, comfort, and peace. I don't know what each day ahead will bring us. I only know that I will be more thankful and appreciative to be with my husband every day we have together. It seems that I have been taking this for granted. Funny how our views of life change when something like this comes our way.

You know, if something was to happen and God only knows if or when it will, I will hopefully not regret anything. I am going to make a point of that from here on out.

Thank you for such wonderful support.

Friday, January 15

I've been telling people for a few weeks now how cold the house has been when I've been home. I thought it was just me and that I was just tired. The kids are barely home, and when they are, they are in front of the fireplace and never complained to me that they were cold. I am having someone come tomorrow to check the furnace.

Because it has been so cold here, it made me think of how nice it would be for Kevin to have a Viking's tie blanket. I bet he would like it, and it would make his hospital room seem more like home. I got the pattern and purchased enough material to make two different blankets. One is for Kevin and one for me to have at the hospital when I visit.

I'm waiting right now in the computer room at the Sister Kenny Institute for Kevin to get back from his therapy session. He will be done for the day at 3:00 p.m. We will be having a *big* outing tonight! John and Nancy are coming to visit, and we're going to walk down the hall to the McDonald's restaurant for supper. This will be such a treat for Kevin.

We are hoping that he will be home next week already! Kevin said he is *really* sick of getting yelled at all of the time! The bed monitors are very sensitive, and he said that when he even moves his butt cheek, the buzzer goes off. This alarms the nurses that a patient is trying to get out of bed, and they come running.

Kevin is also *really* sick of being here, the food, and *everything*! Yes, he does know how blessed he is to be here but still wants to be done.

You see, I can't stay overnight with Kevin when he is in SKI, Sister Kenny Institute, and the staff can't have me help Kevin with anything at all either. This is really different for him to have to wait all of the time for staff to come when he needs help. When we were in the ICU and on the eighth floor, the nurses pretty well trusted me and needed me to watch him. It helped that I was always there and I got to know what they expected, so they felt confident that I would call if I had any trouble. All Kevin had to do before he came to SKI is motion to me with his finger, and I knew what he wanted me to get him or do to help him. He didn't even have to ask me, just wave his finger.

It will take some time for Kevin to talk better and stronger as the days go on. As you see, from my e-mail yesterday, he also did speech therapy. From only a whisper on Sunday to how strong he is today is so amazing.

I want you to know how much I appreciate you reading this. I feel that every time I write, you are hearing me and praying for me. I find this very personal and something that I can reply at anytime to anyone of you and you would be there and understand as to what's happening. Thanks!

This is the second night in a row that I haven't been able to spend the night with Kevin. I miss him so much!

SATURDAY, JANUARY 16
(update typed SUNDAY, JANUARY 17, 5:38 A.M.)

The Sister Kenny Institute has a beautician/barber who is available for shaving and hair care. Early this morning, Kevin had his beard and mustache, which he grew while being here, shaved *off*. He also had his hair cut.

Kevin called me when he was able to during a therapy break this morning. He had told me that he only slept three to four hours last night. He was restless and had a difficult night. He told me that the doctors gave him a CT scan already this morning. They were concerned with how rapid his heart rate was. I wasn't too concerned about this news because I thought that his rate increase was due to his intense therapy schedule. I was relieved and pleased, however, that the doctors wanted to make sure that there are no underlying issues with this change of Kevin's vitals. He also told me how good he is doing in therapy and that the nurses are surprised of how quickly his strength is coming back.

After the phone call, I continued with my goals for the day. I was making a dessert and meals for the kids, doing bills, and cleaning the house. I had a plan of what I needed to do before my return to the hospital to be with Kevin.

Meanwhile, my brother-in-law, John, had come over to start putting the necessary rails up. He was also there to meet with the repairman and me in regard to checking the furnace. I needed him there to help me with the decision of what to do. They checked it out and informed me that our furnace was broken. As soon as they told me this, the phone started ringing. While I went to answer the phone, my mind was racing. I thought, *No wonder, it was freezing in this house! Now what? What else is going to go wrong? How are we going to pay for this? Did this do any damage to the house pipes? What is Kevin going to say? Is this going to worry him more?*

When I answered the phone, my heart began sinking instantly when I found out it was the Sister Kenny Institute. They told me that Kevin needed to go back to the hospital as soon as possible. They found a clot from the CT scan this morning that is on his right lung. He needed to be moved to where the medical staff is more aware and capable of treating this clot. I got flustered, concerned, and upset at this news. I felt like my mind was going a million miles an hour.

The first thing that I had thought of was that Kevin had been complaining of a sore spot on the right side of his stomach. This had started hurting him ever since he woke up in the ICU six days ago. The doctors, Kevin, and I were thinking that it was a sore spot from the blood-thinner shots at the time. He had been receiving these shots in his belly during the whole time that he was in his sedated mode.

Now what is this clot? How serious is this? How scared is Kevin? I wondered what is going through his mind also.

I instantly asked my brother-in-law, John, and the repairman to handle everything with the furnace themselves. I trusted whatever they decided to do. I quickly got my overnight bag and drove to the hospital as fast as I could.

On the way to the hospital, I had called my friends, Jill and Dede, and sister, Penny. I needed them to come over and finish what I had been working on because I didn't know how long I would be gone at this point. The baking wasn't done, and I had everything scattered around the kitchen and house yet. The kids weren't home to finish this for me either.

When I arrived in Kevin's room on the fifth floor, I was stunned to see him. Wow! Kevin looks ten years younger than me now. Not only has he lost quite a bit of weight, but I didn't realize how different just a shave and cut would make. He looks so sexy!

A short while later, the nurse came in and was able to visit with us about what their concerns were at this time.

Kevin and I were very scared, of course, when we had first heard what she had all told us. We were also a little bit relieved when we heard of how common it is to develop a blood clot when a patient has been bedridden for such a long time. This clot is still something to be concerned with, but we are praying that it will go away in time with prayers and medication.

There are again no visitors, phone calls, or anything today until Kevin gets evaluated and treated.

Again, I am able to stay by Kevin's side in the hospital, day and night, which is very helpful for Kevin's healing. Our spirits are better now that we are here together.

Kevin was getting anxious again in the early evening and in need of doing something and get out of his room. We walked to the elevator and back. When we got back, the nurse checked on him, and his heart rate was 124 when it should have been from 95 to 100. He was told that he can only walk across the hall to the family room to watch TV until he is cleared of this clot. They can't take any chances with him anymore.

He is currently on heparin, which is a form of blood thinner and will change to the Coumadin medicine tomorrow.

Kevin is currently on the fifth floor of Abbott NW Hospital until the clot is gone and the doctors are sure they have him on the right dose of Coumadin.

In the early evening, Tony called. All I could hear was screaming. Tony said, "What do I do? The girls are pulling each other's hair, screaming and hitting each other! They won't stop!" I asked him, "Is anyone bleeding yet?" He said "no". I told him that he needed to tell the girls what he wants them to do and then go downstairs. Leave them fight it out. If they need you, they will come get you.

Evidentially it worked because everything was back to normal before we went to sleep for the night. This made us very aware that the kids needed us now. They have been alone without enough parental support and presence for too long of a time now. We need to get Kevin better and back home. The stress of Kevin's illness is very apparent on all of the kids also.

We are hoping and praying that everything goes Kevin's way and that Sister Kenny will discharge him from the fifth floor. It would be so nice to have him come home for outpatient therapy instead of going back to the institute for therapy review and discharge.

I've been told by others that there will be good days and bad days ahead. I think that we all feel at times that there are good days and bad days in daily life period. I really don't know what to expect or what the future days will hold. Nobody does. Only God does, but I'm sure there will be days I will need to ask for help, be sad, etc.

I do feel, however, that if I look at a day that's not going my way and say, "Wow, I'm glad that part's over with" or "God doesn't give us more than we can handle" or "I'm glad I was able to be here to help," even if I would just look for something good that will come out of the situation, all days would be classified as pretty good or just plain good or great. This is me asking each one of you to remind me nicely of what I just wrote, if you feel the need. At the time, I might look at you funny but will think about it and change my mind.

Kevin and I are both really excited that the kids are coming to the hospital tomorrow to watch the football game with us. They haven't been able to see Kevin very often due to sporting, school and church schedules and how he had been feeling.

You are a blessing to me for being my partner in prayer and concern and love for Kevin.

SUNDAY, JANUARY 17, 6:23 P.M.

Kevin had a fair night last night. His blood pressure and heart rate were high again all day today. His potassium and magnesium levels were low this morning, and he was given meds for this.

We both were very anxious to have the three kids come to the hospital today. We decided to make this gathering a football party. I had told a number of other patients that we have met during our stay that they were more than welcome to join in on the feast. I had asked the kids to bring some food from home, and we also received a package of some food from one of Kevin's old classmate's sister, Robyn. I will try to make this relaxing and will try to make it just as if we were home together.

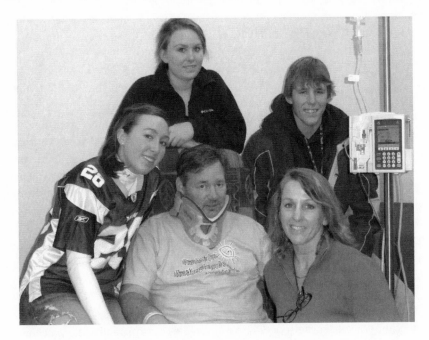

Pictured here from left to right. Front: Kaylee,
Kevin, and Karen. Back: Stephanie and Tony.

This time came and went very quickly. It was really sad to say good-bye to the kids and send them on their way home again. I know that they felt comfort in seeing Kevin out of bed and talking.

Out of nowhere, a man whom I had never met before walked into the room we were resting in. Kevin's eyes lit up, and the biggest smile came over his face. It was Todd, a friend of his from school. They hadn't seen each other in so many years, yet it seemed like it was just yesterday that they visited. It was really nice for both of us.

In the early evening, we were told that Kevin would need an echocardiogram tomorrow. The doctors want to see if there was a blood clot on his heart due to his high pulse. Kevin's pulse was running from 100 to 110. His normal count is 70. Oh, my God, what's next? Now there's a blood clot on his heart? This is bad! Once again, we looked at each other in disbelief. There were so many thoughts that raced through our minds. What does this mean? How serious could this be? I was really sad, scared, and disappointed.

I called my mom, and I had told her of my concern. She told me that God's been with us this far and that he won't leave us now. I knew that was true, but what happened to God's will be done? What is his will for Kevin?

Kevin and I were both extremely concerned and stunned at this news. We couldn't do anything about it, so we just went to sleep with prayer on our minds. Deep down, I was thinking that, sure, tomorrow will come and we won't get the test taken until later in the day again. We will have to wait again and not know the answer again right away but just wait, wait, wait.

MONDAY, JANUARY 18, 4:37 P.M.

Kevin doesn't sleep well here at all. He gets so uncomfortable from the sticky garments and sheets. He has been sweating through his clothing and sheets an average of three times per night. The bed is also very sensitive to any movement. This bed on the fifth floor not only alarms the nurses, but it also makes sounds whenever you move too. I think it's like his leg braces that filled with air. This must help to stimulate your body while lying down.

At 8:30 a.m., the doctor came to do the test on Kevin. When he was done, he told us that the doctors will inform us of the results either later on today or tomorrow. Wait, wait, wait, wait. A little later, medical staff did come in and informed us that there was nothing that they saw on the testing that was abnormal at this time.

What a relief! Where did the spot or clot go? I exhaled a sigh of relief and thanked God for answering my prayers again. Just then, I turned around in my chair and asked Kevin, "How are your spirits today?" He was sleeping really sound while watching the cooking show that he loves so much. I think he was very relieved at the results too and is exhausted.

So far, we've been in the hospital for twenty-eight days. Good thing, Kevin wasn't awake for most of it. He can't get out of here and back home soon enough.

Thank you for keeping us in your prayers. I know that God fixed the problems that we've faced here.

TUESDAY, JANUARY 19, 5:26 P.M., FIRST E-MAIL

Can you believe it? It seems like we might be coming home today. We are still just waiting and hoping that nothing comes up again that would keep us here again. I am of mixed emotions with this. I know you are probably saying, "What? This is what you all were hoping for!"

You know, I'm overly exceedingly glad to have our family together again. I will be happy that Kevin will be home and glad to be able to sleep in a bed instead of chairs, a couch, and a recliner that doesn't recline.

On the other hand, I also will now be in charge of Kevin's health with no help from the nurses at all now. I am scared and insecure. Yes, even after all of the positive miracles that have happened. I will keep you informed of his progress as we go on from this point of his illness.

Thank you for your prayers, concern, gifts of friendship, and gifts to help in any way necessary.

Chapter 5

HOME AND THE NEXT STEP

We got the good news in the early evening that we can go home! We wanted to surprise the kids, so we didn't tell anyone we were able to leave the hospital at this time. We were able to get a wheelchair for Kevin before we left the hospital. The bad thing is they didn't have a wheelchair with a head support on it, and Kevin's neck is weak and gets sore and tired quickly. We were told that I could exchange it for a different one in Buffalo this week.

The drive home was amazing. It was dark, and we were conversing about how we were going to surprise the kids. When we got home, the kids weren't used to me coming home with Kevin. What a surprise! The kids were so happy. It was so nice to be together again! Kevin sat on his couch in the same spot that he always sits and looked so much more satisfied. We were well aware of the challenges ahead of us all. Challenges like bathing, traveling to the doctor appointments, and getting his strength back.

We are very fortunate that at this time, I currently only work out of the house in the fall season. This allows me to be with Kevin and care for him 24/7. Because of this, I was also able to be with Kevin most of the days he was hospitalized. If I hadn't been there to help the nurses and doctors, they wouldn't have let him leave the hospital with me yet. It will be tough at first trying to reorganize family *and* Kevin together again. With the grace of God, it will get done.

I have been told a number of times that nobody knows the future, so trust in the Lord and put everything at the foot of the cross. I really have been trying and would like to ask you to pray for me on that aspect also.

I need to give Kevin shots of heparin, which is a blood thinner, in the stomach twice a day. All I can tell you is that it sure isn't like giving a horse a shot! There is no fur to hide the visibility of the needle going into the skin like it is for an animal. Kevin watches me the whole time and instructs me where to stick the needle. This makes me feel like he doesn't have faith in me that I will do it right. Oh, well, I guess I would do that too if it was me.

Kevin has been very tired and doesn't sleep very well. He doesn't have much of an appetite yet, but we know this will all change with time.

Words can't say enough of how we feel about the kindness, prayers, support, and unity we have received already and know it will be there as we tread ahead with this illness.

WEDNESDAY, JANUARY 20

I knew that I would need to give Kevin a bath and care for his every need. The doctors told me he's not to be left alone at all. We were allowed to take Kevin's brace off for bathing only. Our shower stall is too small to fit a chair in, so Kevin needed to get in the bathtub. This was a much easier task with use of the rails that John installed. I washed his hair with a cup so he wouldn't need to bend his neck, and then I washed his body.

When Kevin gets stronger, he should be able to stand in the shower. I made sure that I didn't preoccupy myself with anything that would take my attention off Kevin. I just wanted him to get used to being home again and make sure that he behaved and used the walker. I was instructed to follow behind Kevin while he used his walker. This was a safety precaution so that in case he starts to fall backward, I can catch him. He isn't steady on his feet yet and needs more strength to be on his own.

THURSDAY, JANUARY 21, 12:48 P.M.

Today was a big day for Kevin. We went to Buffalo to do some errands. He was *very* anxious to get out of the house, and the doctors told us that he needs to try to walk daily. Kevin walked with me through Menards today just to pick up a few things. I don't think he realized how hard this was going to be. I could see how hard Kevin was trying and saw a look of disappointment in his eyes. He didn't want to quit but knew that he was done walking in stores for the rest of the day. He did his best.

Kevin was content to wait for me in the truck as I finished some other stops that we needed to do. We picked up a walker and replaced the current wheelchair we have for one with a neck support. We are planning on only using the wheelchair for sporting events and church. These are times that he will need to sit and have more neck support. When we are out and about, we will use Kevin's walker and/or the shopping cart for stabilization.

Kevin had a doctor appointment today also for his blood test. This visit went well. We were told that we could quit the Coumadin shots completely and reduce the intake of the Coumadin meds, which is blood thinner.

You know, as far as the shots go, Kevin told me it hurt when I pushed the needle harder into his skin while dispensing, when I was too far away from his belly button, etc. I really tried to improve my technique and I think I got pretty good. Even the doctor said today that he's seen quite a bit more bruising on other patients, and Kevin only had three or four pink dots. Hey, I was just getting *really good*! I almost perfected it, and now, I have to quit. I am just kidding!

Kevin wanted to go to work but knew that he would be too weak to get out of the truck. As soon as we arrived at work, I went in and told everyone I saw that Kevin was in the truck. His brothers and cousins came out to see him. I could see the happiness that they felt to be with their brother and co-worker again. They were able to talk about business and update Kevin on the goings-on in the company for a short time. I think that if we can stop by the office a few times each week, this will really be a good boost for Kevin. It gave him some normality in his day-to-day activities.

We are so happy that Kevin is home. Still as I go through the day, there are times that I am doing my thing and all of a sudden start to cry. Is it sadness? Is it tears of happiness? Is it reliving the past month in my mind? What a miracle it is that Kevin is alive and with us today! There has been so much that has happened and so many different emotions. How can you pinpoint even just one of these? I have been told that this is a normal reaction and will still continue from time to time.

In the evening, we planned on attending the basketball game. When we arrived at the school and made our way to the gym, the principal showed us a good place for us to be during the game. Being as Kevin is in the wheelchair, we were told to sit on the opposite side of the gym. This gave Kevin great visibility of the game and allowed us to be out of the way of fan traffic.

Friends and well-wishers still came over to visit with Kevin and me when they could. It was so nice. It was like everyone took turns so Kevin wouldn't be overwhelmed. People were genuinely concerned with our whole family's well-being and offered continued prayers for us. It was good to see Kevin smiling and greeting friends and wonderful to watch the girls play too.

We know that we unfortunately still missed talking to a lot of people but know that as Kevin gets stronger, we will get another chance.

Take care and God bless each and every one of you!

FRIDAY, JANUARY 22, 7:39 P.M.

I can tell you that Kevin *doesn't* like it when I drive. He never has liked being a passenger in a vehicle and especially now. I need to drive down toward the cities more than ever with him for doctor appointments and feel that I'm doing a good job. I'm getting used to it and trying to ignore his comments.

Kevin had another doctor appointment this morning in Buffalo to check his blood level. It's interesting to find out all of the details that go into getting the right dose of Coumadin levels. Kevin's blood is a little thin so they are going to reduce the amount of medications.

We've been going places each day, and he has been able to get time to walk here and there. We've got to keep him in shape so he is strong when he goes to the Mayo Clinic this summer. It's like at home, I wait to hear the sound of the walker being set on the kitchen floor and the wheels rolling along with the two back legs of the walker pads, dragging along after. This alerts me to pay attention to the steady sound of movement and helps me know where he is at all times. I am able to watch as Kevin puts his weight on it as he walks slowly to his destination.

It was very hard for me to put the wheelchair in and out of the back of the Suburban. Kevin's cousin, Gary, put together a system using plywood that I have been using that is easier on my back. It took a while to get the hang of it, but it works for me.

Kevin still has been tired, especially at night, and still isn't able to sleep well. The doctor did tell him that it might take a few months before he will get a good night's sleep.

At the basketball game, David, who I found out is a cancer survivor himself, visited with us. He made a *great* point that we need to remember. He said, "A good and positive attitude is very important when faced with an illness. Kevin may have 40 percent of his bone marrow infected with cancer, but he also has 60 percent cancer-free."

Kevin needs to go to the blood doctor at Buffalo for Coumadin level testing three times per week.

Next Wednesday, January 27, he goes for x-rays and a visit with his surgeon and then goes to Waconia for radiation testing. He will start radiation February 1 and will need fifteen treatments, have two weeks off, and then go to the Mayo Clinic for a pilot program. I don't have any details yet as to what the pilot program consists of or what they will be doing. I'm sure I will find out when they have information as to how the cancer is reacting to radiation.

I still cry at times but don't always feel bad when I cry. I can describe it as a humbling feeling. I looked up what humbling meant in the dictionary, and it means submissive.

I know Kevin is in God's hands and I have been very excited to show everyone proof of one of God's miracles that we have experienced. Kevin's scar looks like it has been healing for four months, not one month. Kevin told me last night after the basketball game that I really don't need to show everyone his scar anymore. The people that have seen it will tell others the proof of the miracle.

I will continue to update you all on Kevin's progress when there are any changes or I have any new information.

I would like to ask you to please continue to pray for Kevin, Kaylee, Tony, Stephanie, friends, family, and myself for strength, trust, and faith.

SATURDAY, JANUARY 23

There were basketball finals in Cokato today, and we both really wanted to go. This will give us a chance to have people in the community see that we are okay and have fun supporting our school at the same time.

We are getting used to using the wheelchair and the schools have been very good about accommodating us. We have always been able to find a spot to sit during the game and still get a good view of the whole floor without Kevin needing to turn his head because he can't.

Sunday, January 24

We went to church, and Kevin was *really* sore but wanted to go to church to praise God in his house and thank him not only for the miracles he has shown us but for everything.

After the service, we were asked if we would like to be prayed over. Kevin had said that he wanted to do this. A large group of parishioner's came to the front of the church, and we all prayed together for healing. A lot of times, others know just what to say in prayer when we have needs, feelings, etc., and we don't know how to put them all in words ourselves. I felt that my concerns, hopes, and desires were all covered with this prayer session. God was using others to pray for me. We also are very grateful for all of the prayers and know they will continue as we travel on this journey of healing.

Monday, January 25

This was a *huge* day for us. It meant so much to Stephanie that Kevin was home for the big game tonight. It was parents' night for the girls' basketball. We didn't stay too long because Kevin got really tired. That's one thing I have to say when he says he's tired and it's time to go, he isn't kidding.

It again was so nice to see everyone and visit with them while hearing positive feedback and hopes of others. Kevin told me when we got home that seeing others and visiting with each person has been very therapeutic for him. He is touched by everyone's concern, prayers, well wishes, and jokes.

Tuesday, January 26, 5:25 p.m.

Last week Kevin had gone to a basketball game, on Thursday and Friday, and a couple on Saturday too. I think this was too much for him even with the use of a wheelchair. All I know is it's *cold* outside. I'm starting to get better in transporting the wheelchair back and forth.

Kevin has been bothered quite a bit lately about his short attention span. This is something new for him because he always has been very attentive, on top of everything and focuses on the topic at hand.

Today we stayed home because he has three doctor appointments tomorrow and he needs to rest.

Kevin still has high spirits and a positive attitude. He thanks the good Lord daily for another day of life. Kevin is a Christian who doesn't usually display his faith publically. He doesn't push his feelings or beliefs on anyone because he feels everyone has a choice. Kevin and I both feel that a person doesn't have to thank God in public or show or tell others that they are praying in order to be a Christian.

Through the miracles that we have been shown, we feel that God is using Kevin as proof to others of his love for us. From the beginning of Kevin's illness, I had a strong desire to share my beliefs through e-mail updates. Usually Kevin wouldn't want me sharing so much personal information to others. He has given approval and has joined me in sharing our faith story in hopes that it might help someone believe in God.

Thank you for being here for us.

WEDNESDAY, JANUARY 27, 4:22 P.M.

Today, Kevin had x-rays and two doctor appointments.

The x-rays were reviewed by the neurosurgeon, and he told us that everything looked fine right now. Dr. Garner understands the urgency of radiation treatment, but wants the bone in Kevin's neck to heal better first. Kevin was hoping that today Dr. Garner would tell him that he no longer needed to wear this neck brace. It's so uncomfortable and hot. Instead, he told us that when radiation treatment starts, he is to wear the neck brace at all times. The only time he can take it off is when he is lying back in the recliner or in bed. This is a caution because the bones could become weaker during radiation, which could cause great injury.

We also had an appointment with a different oncologist in Waconia who explained just a few more things to us.

I was incorrect on the date that radiation will start. On February 1, Kevin has an appointment with radiation. He still won't be receiving radiation on this visit. Instead, this will be a time for him to get a consult, his first simulation, planning session, and radiation-planning CT scan. Kevin's radiation will start February 8 and will be Monday through Friday for three weeks.

I will be scheduling and getting information on the Mayo Clinic appointments today.

It's important to Kevin not to miss many of the kid's sporting events if possible. It's not possible for Kevin to go to Kaylee's softball games yet. The practices and the games take longer than he can take.

We want to extend our many thanks for the prayers of healing and comfort that you have given to me and our family.

MONDAY, FEBRUARY 1

Kevin had his simulation appointment in Waconia today. Simulation is a process used to plan radiation therapy. They plan where the target area that they need to radiate is precisely located. When the target area is located, they mark it first on Kevin's neck and then on a mold. Each patient has their own mold perfected for them to use so each time it is exact. In order for the mold to be made, Kevin had to hold his head and neck in an uncomfortable position for half an hour. This was very hard for him to do, and it made him *very* sore.

The following appointments that follow won't be nearly as long, so it shouldn't bother his neck again.

The completed mold will have breathing holes and be placed on Kevin's head when he has radiation treatments. It will be secured to the table during radiation so there is no chance for any movement at all.

TUESDAY, FEBRUARY 2

The doctors felt that Kevin needed more radiation. He had his first radiation treatment today and will now have treatment Monday through Friday for four weeks instead of three.

At times, there are side effects because radiation kills bad cells but also damage good cells. These side effects usually don't start, if ever, for two to three weeks after treatment begins and could last four to six weeks after treatment ends. Kevin *could* experience fatigue; mouth changes; hoarse voice; sores; dry mouth; loss of taste; tooth decay; changes in taste; infections of gums, teeth, or tongue; jaw stiffness; bone changes; and skin changes. Esophagitis could also occur. Esophagitis is when the throat becomes inflamed and sore.

Kevin's spirits are *very* positive and *really* doing well with the change of his daily life. He really doesn't like staying home from work. He feels like he can't do anything but knows he doesn't have a choice right now.

It would be different for Kevin if his cancer would have just stayed in his bone marrow and wouldn't have grown a tumor that ate his vertebrae. He wouldn't be so restricted because he wouldn't have needed any surgery. When you think about it, if Kevin's neck wouldn't have been so sore and numb, how long would it have taken for us to find out that he has cancer? How long would it have taken us to go to the doctor? What stage would this cancer have to be for us to notice that something was wrong? What would have warned us? How would we have known? It doesn't seem like it, but this was a blessing for us. This is also a warning for all of us to take care of the bodies we have been given. Notice any changes in our bodies and get them taken care of.

I listed the side effects so you all could pray against them and that Kevin won't get any of them. The power of prayer and love that we have received has been so evident and strong. I think about this often and am in awe, thankful and humble.

These updates that I have been doing have been very therapeutic for me. Not only has this helped me, but it also has brought people together in prayer, in memory, and in long-lost friendship. Kevin's friend and classmate, Mike, has created an e-mail list of classmates. When he gets an e-mail update from our friend Al or Patti, he forwards them all to his classmates. They too have e-mailed Kevin and sent well wishes via cards, phone calls, and visits. Kevin even received a gift of a game I guess they used to play in their younger years. This has all meant so much to him.

Thank you again for everything.

MONDAY, FEBRUARY 8, 1:59 P.M.

Kevin has had four radiation treatments this past week. The treatments don't hurt at all, but Kevin is *very* tired.

70

His blood-thinner medicine has been stable, and it doesn't need to be checked again for two weeks.

Kevin has been having visitors and enjoying them very much.

We had our Erickson Christmas party yesterday at our home, which was so much fun. We made our annual Swedish dish called Kroppkaka and ate too much food. Kevin, of course, is very tired today. I figure that we will do as much as possible now like visiting and going to games just in case he starts not feeling well in a couple of weeks.

Hopefully, we will hear from the Mayo Clinic tomorrow as to the treatment schedule we will have when we go there in March.

I found out Friday that the doctors in Waconia who are doing the radiation will not be checking on how the cancer is reacting to this radiation. I don't like that. How do we know that this really killed the tumor or not? We will find that out I guess when we go to the Mayo Clinic.

You remember when I wrote that we shouldn't take life for granted? How we need to appreciate loved ones and make time for them? Well, I sure blew that! As soon as Kevin came home from the hospital, my blinders went on again. I was trying to tackle all of the things that I need to do, leaving no time for Kevin. I mean, special time, even if it is having a cup of coffee with him. I am so glad that I have caught myself now and have the opportunity to start fresh again.

Thank you for your thoughts and prayers.

THURSDAY, FEBRUARY 11

It is Tony's senior year, and it was so wonderful that Kevin was able to watch the game tonight. It was Parents' Night, and we both were able to support him.

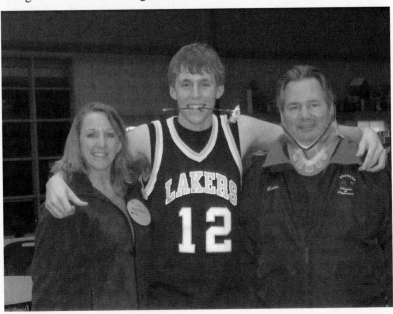

SATURDAY, FEBRUARY 13, 9:53 P.M.

Kevin has had nine out of twenty radiation treatments so far. He has *not* had any side effects from this so far other than thicker saliva.

Today, Kevin doesn't feel very good at all but thinks he is getting a cold, so we are staying put this weekend.

We are *very* fortunate to have you all for support during this time. It sure feels like this is going on for *a long* time. Thank you for your concern, kindness, and prayers for us and our families.

SUNDAY, FEBRUARY 14, 8:07 P.M.

It's Valentine's Day today. I am so happy and blessed to have the love of my life still with me. We don't do the gift or date thing because we feel that Valentine's Day is just another day. We should show love and make *each* day as special as the next. I'm feeling very emotional today maybe because I'm tired or have tears of happiness that we are together.

I hope you don't mind, but these e-mails are therapy for me, and sometimes people respond with just the right thing to say to get me straight and remind me of my faith.

I was sent the following story from my friend, Steve. This touched me so much.

The Quilt Holes'

As I faced my Maker at the last judgment, I knelt before the Lord along with all the other souls. Before each of us laid our lives like the squares of a quilt in many piles; an angel sat before each of us sewing our quilt squares together into a tapestry that is our life.

But as my angel took each piece of cloth off the pile, I noticed how ragged and empty each of my squares was. They were filled with giant holes. Each square was labeled with a part of my life that had been difficult, the challenges and temptations I was faced with in everyday life. I saw hardships that I endured, which were the largest holes of all.

I glanced around me. Nobody else had such squares. Other than a tiny hole here and there, the other tapestries were filled with rich color and the bright hues of worldly fortune. I gazed upon my own life and was disheartened.

My angel was sewing the ragged pieces of cloth together, threadbare and empty, like binding air.

Finally the time came when each life was to be displayed, held up to the light, the scrutiny of truth. The others rose; each in turn, holding up their tapestries. So filled their lives had been. My angel looked upon me and nodded for me to rise.

My gaze dropped to the ground in shame. I hadn't had all the earthly fortunes. I had love in my life and laughter. But there had also been trials of illness and wealth, and false accusations that took from me my world, as I knew it. I had to start over many times. I often struggled with the temptation to quit, only to somehow muster the strength to pick up and begin again. I spent many nights on my knees in prayer, asking for help and guidance in my life. I had often been held up to ridicule, which I endured painfully, each time offering it up to the Father in hopes that I would not melt within my skin beneath the judgmental gaze of those who unfairly judged me.

And now, I had to face the truth! My life was what it was, and I had to accept it for what it was.

I rose and slowly lifted the combined squares of my life to the light.

An awe-filled gasp filled the air. I gazed around at the others who stared at me with wide eyes.

Then, I looked upon the tapestry before me. Light flooded the many holes, creating an image, the face of Christ. Then our Lord stood before me, with warmth and love in His eyes. He said, 'Every time you gave over your life to Me it became My life, My hardships, and My struggles.

Each point of light in your life is when you stepped aside and let Me shine through, until there was more of Me than there was of you.'

May all our quilts be threadbare and worn, allowing Christ to shine through!

Sometimes it's hard to put our pains at the foot of the cross. It hurts me to see Kevin going through all of this and have asked God why him and not me? I mean, I am the one with all of the physical issues. I seem to be weaker now, both physically and emotionally, than when Kevin was in the hospital. I don't know why.

I too, like most of you, have had other trials in my life. I don't remember for a fact that I gave them all to God to take care of but know that he took care of them anyway for me because he loves me and he loves you too.

I want a quilt with many holes and will put Kevin in God's hands. I will need to read this story from time to time to remind myself of this.

Thank you for reading this and I hope this helps you too.

TUESDAY, FEBRUARY 16

It's my birthday today. Kevin made me a poached egg on toast for breakfast. I loved it; it tasted so good. I even took a nap in the afternoon, which I *never do*! Then I got to pick TV movies for the night and relaxed. It was a great day. It made me feel good to have someone take care of me today.

WEDNESDAY, FEBRUARY 17

After Kevin's doctor appointment, we went to Buffalo, and I ran into my friend, Kim. She wanted to know if I had opened her e-mail message that she had sent me for my birthday yet. She seemed so disappointed that I hadn't opened my e-mail at all, so when I got home, I sat by the computer to read it. I couldn't believe it! There were so many well wishes that I had received on my birthday and I didn't even realize it.

I asked Kevin, "How in the world does everyone know it was my birthday? Even your classmates from Golden Valley school knew." I just couldn't figure it out.

That night, at church, Kim spilled the beans to me that she had Al forward to everyone on the list that it was my birthday. Right after that, Nita came up to me and wished me happy birthday too. I asked her how she knew, and she told me it was in the newspaper. I couldn't believe it was in the newspaper too! When we came home, Kevin found it. Sure enough! Thank you, Sheri! Thank you for your thoughts and kindness. I really felt special with all of this attention.

Now for Kevin, I can't take the whole spotlight, you know. Kevin's only side effect so far from his radiation is his skin on his neck is getting something rashlike. We put aloe vera on it a couple times a day. The doctor said that if he hasn't gotten a sore throat already, he probably won't get one.

The other good news is Kevin's blood-thinner medicine, Coumadin, is still regulated well.

THURSDAY, FEBRUARY 18

It's hard for me to see Kevin getting weaker. It's tough to watch him walk away from me for treatment at the radiation appointments. I want to take it all away from him. I want to take his place. If only it was me instead.

Family members are allowed to watch loved ones receive the radiation treatment just one time. The other times, I need to wait in the waiting room and visit with other caregivers and patients or just wait and read.

Well, today was the day I was asked to watch this take place. I kind of knew what to expect because we were given information explaining this whole procedure before Kevin even did his first one. I also saw pictures, and we talked about it. I realized today that reading about it and seeing pictures of it doesn't cut it. It's nothing like seeing your loved one actually being treated. I didn't do very well with this at all!

Kevin laid on the table, and the nurses put the mesh mask mold on his head and attached it to the table. Then they measured and adjusted the machine to the exact location for the radiation to begin. Kevin couldn't move his head even if he wanted to. He was locked in. This is a safety issue and something that is necessary, but at the same time, he looked helpless.

This reminded me of Kevin being in the hospital bed with medical staff around him while he was restrained and helpless. It seemed as if I was waiting for him to get agitated or feel claustrophobic, but he didn't. He was motionless. I started to cry to myself and then it hit me again. *Oh my God! Kevin has cancer!*

Once they had Kevin in place and locked on the table, we all needed to leave. Nobody can be in the room when the radiation is turned on.

When the nurses told me that we had to leave, it reminded me of when the nurses told me that I needed to leave in the hospital. When I needed to leave because he was getting agitated and restless and I couldn't help him get off of his restraints.

I felt helpless once again, wishing that I could get him out.

The control room where the nurses conducted the radiation was very impressive. I, of course, didn't understand a thing that they said. We watched the treatment from a camera in the control room and were able to see how this machine worked and understood why it didn't take long to perform. The machine went from one side of the neck, did radiation, turned around to the other side and did radiation again, and that was it. The radiation was turned off, and the staff went in and got Kevin out.

Every Thursday we meet with the doctor at the radiation clinic after his treatment. During this time, we receive any new information and are able to ask questions. After Kevin's treatment today, I was sent to the meeting room ahead of Kevin. I was still crying and upset when Kevin came in the room. He couldn't understand why I was crying, but when I explained it, he had a blank look on his face. Was he trying to remember how it felt to be tied down? Does he even remember? I don't think he even remembers. It's hard to explain this to him. Sometimes it's hard for someone to imagine unless you've been there yourself.

The doctor arrived, and I had pulled myself together just in time. We were talked to about the blood tests that were done the week before to check on the blood count, etc. There wasn't anything that the doctors feel is abnormal for this condition at this time.

Kevin said, other than the neck issues, he feels like he doesn't even have cancer. He just gets a little more tired at the end of the day than he usually did. This goes to show and remind everyone that we all need to pay attention when even the smallest change or ache happens because not everything is obvious.

The last radiation treatment is Monday, March 1. Tuesday, March 2, we will be at the Mayo Clinic in Rochester for consultation and testing. It will take two to four days of testing. When they have the results of the tests read, they will decide what treatment they want Kevin to have.

I am very anxious for this time because I am in need of some answers again and will be praying for good ones.

Thanks for being my buddies.

Chapter 6

MAYO TESTING AND PLAN OF ACTION

TUESDAY, MARCH 2

Today is our first day at the Mayo Clinic in Rochester. We met with Dr. Russel today for a consultation and plan for the week. The doctor gave Kevin a thorough exam and asked about all of his past sicknesses, hospitalizations, and family history. There was nothing out of the ordinary in Kevin's past, but the doctor directed his questions to his high blood pressure and high triglycerates. Dr. Russel said, "Kevin, you sure had a dramatic entrance to the Multiple Myeloma disease!"

We were told that this disease shuts down all other fighting cells in the system, so illnesses can happen *very* easily. Not only can this cancer cause kidney problems, but it is *very important* that Kevin doesn't come in contact with *any* sickness or bacteria! This could interfere with the cancer treatment.

Today, after visiting with Dr. Russel, Kevin was given a schedule of places and times that we needed to go to for testing from now until Friday, here at the Mayo. Kevin had a urine test, a blood test, and a chest x-ray today and was also given another urine test jug to do for twenty-four hours.

WEDNESDAY, MARCH 3

At 8:15 a.m., Kevin had a bone marrow collection test. This test will give the current percentage of cancer in the bone marrow and possibly tell the doctors other important information also.

Kevin is *really* tired and sore on his lower back, where they took marrow out of.

It's *amazing* how wonderful and organized this hospital is.

Kevin's spirits are really good! He has the right attitude, whereas I am having a more emotional time. I think that when we find out the treatment plan and a more updated report of the cancer, I will feel better. I do know and have read over and over about how I need to put this all at the foot of the cross and let God handle this, but I just feel like my heart is broken and needs repair.

Kevin isn't going to have a spinal check down here because the doctors are concerned that the surgery hasn't been that long ago. They realized also that he already has an appointment scheduled next week to see the surgeon to check on it anyway. Because this saved us another doctor appointment down here, we will be coming home already today sometime.

My family physician referred me to the Mayo Clinic in October 2009, for my health issues. I was declined due to the wide range of testing and availability of time needed for head traumas. I decided to try to get a new referral from my neurology specialist back home this time. I had to cancel my previous appointment for this consult because we had conflicts with Kevin's doctor appointments and his were more necessary than mine at the time. I received a call yesterday by my specialist back home to see if I could come in for an appointment due to a cancellation from a patient. I had turned it down because we were in Rochester and had appointments. Well, today, when we found out that we were coming home for a day, I called, and they *still had an opening*! I was very happy about that and was hoping that this will help me get a closer step to coming here too.

We will need to come back for three more appointments for Kevin on Friday. We will find out at that time the results from the tests that have been done and what treatment plan will need to be done. I, again, will e-mail updates ASAP.

I'm so very thankful to Al and Patti for the time they've put into creating the e-mail lists. This allows so many friends and family members to know the same facts as everyone else.

FRIDAY, MARCH 5, 11:00 P.M.

Today we met with two doctors at the Mayo Clinic to review the test results from earlier in the week. They suggested a treatment plan to start with for this Myeloma cancer.

Dr. Russel said the skeletal x-rays that were taken showed no more bad cells have clumped together creating any more tumors at this time. There is, however, worry for skeletal damage with this disease. There is a monthly/bimonthly infusion that Kevin will start this next Monday at the Mayo Clinic. Infusion therapy strengthens your bones. It is better to start this infusion at the early stages of treatment and will probably continue to do this for two years.

Kevin's blood work shows that he is slightly anemic, but the doctors are hoping to get this up as treatment takes hold. He will need to start taking calcium and vitamin D because his levels were low.

The blood protein level is also important to maintain for his kidney and liver functions. At the current time, the level is fine, but they will keep track of it. The bone marrow extractions showed 25 to 30 percent cancer cell inhabitants at this time. This number is different from the previous test, but we were told that this test can be different each time. It depends on what spot of marrow the test was taken from. There could be pockets that contain more bad cells elsewhere in the marrow. The genetic bone marrow test will determine the level of risk, and the results are not back yet. They are getting Kevin started on his medications now and will change the plan or up the medications if needed after the results are back.

The recommended treatment at this time for killing the cancer is taking Revlimid, which is an oral pill, for twenty-one out of twenty-eight days for four months; dexamethasone, which is an oral pill, one time per week; and a daily pill of Nexium to help prevent acid damage to his stomach. Valcade is a medicine that may be added later on if needed. The side effects from all of these are mood change, appetite, hunger, fluid retention, acid damage to stomach, rash, fatigue, and constipation. These can also cause blood clots, but he is on Coumadin now already anyway. We will find out in a month or two how the Myeloma disease is reacting to the treatment. Isn't medicine amazing?

Then we had an appointment with Dr. Kumar, who talked about the stem cell transplant.

The average success of this transplant is two to three years before reoccurrence. The good thing is that this process can be done again to prolong life. So you see, Kevin is in good hands and even better because of all of the prayers and support from all of our friends.

Today was hard for Kevin because he was informed *by the doctor*, not me telling him, about the possibility of a timetable of life. We are overwhelmed right now but will take each day as it comes.

When we go home, Kevin will continue to get his blood drawn weekly from our local doctor. They will fax the blood test results down to the Mayo Clinic for them to view.

This is just another reminder of how we need to live each day to the fullest. This is *our* chapter in *our* lives right now, but what is yours? Everybody has one.

I keep *trying* to remember to live every day with Kevin to the fullest as I'm sure you do with your loved ones. I know I need to work on this with the kids also, which, as I'm sure you all know, can be trying at times.

Kevin and I were talking and agreed that God may be using him as an inspiration to others who are ill. Kevin is determined to keep going with a good attitude. He always says, "What are you going to do? Life goes on!"

I love this man so much and know we have so much to teach each other, experience together, and learn together yet in our life together. We've only been married for eleven years and plan on being grandparents together.

God's will be done, but I will beg and plead with him to heal Kevin.

Sometimes I feel like I'm whining, but I am letting you know my thoughts, so you can join me in begging God to take this Myeloma away. I pray for healing for all of your needs also.

MONDAY, MARCH 8

Kevin had an appointment at the Mayo Clinic for a procedure called skeletal infusion. I mentioned this in the previous e-mail. It strengthens the bones.

The Multiple Myeloma disease attacks the bones and makes them weak, so he was infused with, what you can call a vitamin, a liquid to put the calcium back in the bone. Isn't that amazing?

There is an infusion with either a three-hour drip or ninety-minute drip. The time difference in the infusion time frame is the speed of the drip. The same amount of medicine is given, but some patients react differently. For example, say if you have arthritis or a different illness that would be affected with a fast drip, you would need the slower three-hour drip. Kevin was scheduled for the ninety-minute drip.

Kevin told me that the only thing that hurt during this procedure was getting poked by the needle. The side effect for this medicine is that in a couple of days after treatment, he might feel like he is getting a cold or flu. He is allowed to take medicine like normal for that.

Guess what! While Kevin was in the room for this, I went to an area that has a baby grand piano. I read earlier that anyone was allowed to play for others at any time. I brought my music and couldn't wait to get that chance. Well, I opened the piano and pulled the music stand toward me and it fell off onto my lap! Oh my God! I couldn't believe it! I tried to put it back on as quietly and quickly as I could but just couldn't manage to do it alone. A nice woman who works at the clinic saw me and came to help me. She said it's happened before and didn't seem alarmed and said just to leave it open when I'm done so it looks inviting for others to play. She loved the music and said it's peaceful for others to hear.

After I finished playing, I went to the cafeteria for lunch. I spotted a couple of handicapped patients that needed help. I felt sorry for them and noticed that nobody else was going to help, so I asked them if they would accept my help. One patient needed his tray carried to his table and food set out for him to eat. I made sure he was seated, and the smile of thanks on his face was rewarding to me. As I was leaving the cafeteria, I noticed an elderly man who was struggling to move with his wheelchair. I had asked him if I could give him a ride. He didn't hesitate to ask me to please take him to his dialysis appointment and directed me to the transfusion department.

That pretty much filled that time for me and made up for my mishap with the piano. This was such a lift for my spirits. I maybe can't help Kevin but am in the right place to feel needed and help others.

We were able to come home after this appointment today and continue care at home.

Chapter 7

CONTINUING ON

Kevin had an upset stomach today, but it went away later on in the day. We figured that this is a possible side effect from his infusion that he had yesterday.

The cancer medicines that Kevin is prescribed to take are only available through the Specialty Pharmacy at the Mayo Clinic. This is due to the fact that these drugs are still in the test mode and are monitored very carefully. Kevin needs to call the Specialty Pharmacy representative each month to answer many questions. The prescriptions will not be sent or refilled unless these questions are answered appropriately. They need to make sure the drugs aren't put in the wrong hands.

It is very important that we time this call for the refill just right. They won't send the medicines early, and you don't want to be late either. If you get the medicines late, you might miss a dose, which in turn could mess up how the drugs are working with the cancer. We are told which day to expect the medications to arrive at our house via FedEx. This way we can make sure that we are home to sign for it. If we're not home, they don't leave them.

We received our first shipment today. Kevin didn't want to start taking them until tonight because we have to get up early tomorrow to go to more doctor appointments. He read that the Revlimid drug will make him tired, so he didn't want to start taking them until later on tonight. He was hoping this would help him get a good night sleep for a change.

I truly see the difficulty Kevin has in regard to getting around. I am fortunate that he is healthy enough to socialize, support our local community, and still enjoy life. The girls' high school basketball team was in the playoffs, and even though it is still really cold, Kevin and I weren't going to miss it.

WEDNESDAY, MARCH 10

Today, Kevin is really tired, and we have two doctor appointments.

The appointment with the surgeon was positive. We were shown the before and after x-ray's of Kevin's surgical spot in his neck. The pictures of the x-rays were amazing and with such detail. It was really good for Kevin to see this because he doesn't remember much of anything from the time of going to urgent care on December 22 to coming out of his induced coma. By seeing the pictures, it explained in better detail to him what they did in surgery. We were given a copy of the CD of the x-rays to take home.

The doctor also explained to us the range of motion that Kevin can expect to achieve. Approval was given for him to start therapy to relieve his muscle tightness and improve his motion. He will start therapy next Monday in Howard Lake and go two times per week for about three weeks.

After the surgeon appointment, we went to Buffalo for his Coumadin check. His level was where the doctor wanted it to be. This too was positive for us because it gave us a feeling of things going our way.

Kevin told me that he definitely wants to get well enough that he can drive his tractor this year yet. He is a determined man that knows what he wants and goes for it. His spirits are good, and we all are waiting patiently for the results of his genetic marrow test to come back yet.

I watch Kevin and can plainly see how happy he is to talk to someone else other than the doctors and me for a change. It seems like he has more energy and excitement during and after conversing with others. The normal teasing hasn't been quite as thick as in the past on both ends. There is so much to talk about, and I think people are being sensitive to Kevin at this time. Kevin wants or needs to get through this and get back to more normality in life. He really needs to get some more crap pretty soon here. We are very thankful for the many greetings from those who have seen us out and about. We are truly blessed to be here in this community.

I have always known that many have it worse than me. It's real easy to forget this from time to time. Because I have medical issues myself, I have seen many with worse arthritis and pain than me. Even in our rural living, I have seen people that can't stand up straight, some who can't move without a limp, some who have lost loved ones, some who have fibromyalgia, and even some who struggle to love others is very painful.

On our first visit to the Mayo, I saw a young woman missing most of her right leg in a wheelchair in the same waiting room as us. She was our age and looked very sad; a very young boy with his head stitched from front to back. I prayed for him to have many years of life left; an infant in a stroller. This infant was being treated for cancer too. How humbling this was!

We all can feel sorry for ourselves at times and think we have it bad. When you really look out of your comfort zone, you will realize that you actually have it good. We need to remember that God doesn't give us anything that we can't handle. Everything is for a reason. We don't and probably won't sometimes understand but giving it all to him is all we can do.

I sure hope I talk the talk and walk the walk more each day as I continue my journey in life. I also will need to be reminded of this often, so I can pass it down to generations to come.

Take care and I will keep in touch with you when things change.

Friday, March 12, 7:52 p.m.

Kevin took his first Revlimid pill Tuesday night and still hasn't seemed to have any side effects from this one yet. This morning, he took his dexamethasone and got so wired he couldn't sit still at all. He was driving me nuts! He finished making my Chow Mein and made Swedish meatballs too. He even heated up my spaghetti I made yesterday for supper and made noodles. Too bad he didn't want to do dishes too.

Being as he was able to do my kitchen work, I was able to finally take down our Christmas decorations.

I visited with a relative and family friend who lost her husband to cancer last year. She is also a nurse at Abbott NW Hospital in the cities. She gave me some well-needed advice. She told me that Kevin and I should do everything together that we can now. Have fun together and explore life. Keep Kevin in shape and talk about important things like his last will while he is still feeling good. The last will is important, because it will let the doctors and me know what his treatment preferences in an end-of-life situation would be. She told me that the road will be tough and I have an open invitation to call her anytime I need. I took this advice very seriously. She knew firsthand all about our journey ahead of us because she was just there herself.

We *still* haven't heard from the Mayo yet as to the outcome of the genetic marrow test. It's always a wait, wait, wait game. Hopefully, we will find out next week.

Take care and God bless!

Saturday, March 13

Our lives are continuing on as close to normal as possible. We are starting to get used to our new routines of doctor appointments and medicines. Kevin has been strong enough to stand in the shower by himself for a little while now. This gives him some independence back, and I'm sure it is much appreciated by him.

Kevin still has a ton of energy again today. He vacuumed the carpet in the living room and cut up celery. It is nice to see him up and about, but I am somewhat concerned about how much he's doing. We were told that this medicine can make you antsy like this.

Monday, March 15, 8:09 a.m.

Kevin woke me up in the middle of the night complaining about tightness in his chest. I got up and the first thing I did was get the list of side effects from the medicines out to read. While going through them, we found out that this could be a side effect. It stated that we should contact our doctor as soon as possible. I had asked Kevin some questions about his pain and the intensity. Guess what?! He told me that this tightness started yesterday, Sunday, afternoon. Come on! Why didn't he tell me at that time? Didn't we learn anything from this whole experience yet? When you feel pain, you need to address it.

I called down to the Mayo Hospital, and they wanted us to come in ASAP. When I informed them that we were three and a half hours away, they directed us to go to Buffalo emergency. The Mayo Clinic was contacted when we arrived at Buffalo. They instructed the medical staff on what tests they wanted performed. They want to make sure that this tightness wasn't caused by a blood clot or anything like that. Thankfully, all of the tests came back good, and we were reassured that everything seemed fine. It's most likely this was just related to the side effects from medicine or possible that Kevin did too much on Saturday. It's hard to stay put when you are agitated and consumed with so much energy.

The doctor at the Mayo Clinic prescribed Kevin to keep taking the current medications. There still could be a side effect of tightness of the chest muscles, but they still wanted no change in dose as of yet.

TUESDAY, MARCH 16, 8:08 A.M.

Kevin has been sleeping *a lot* and didn't feel very good as of last night. Today is another day we can be together, and hopefully, Kevin will feel better when he wakes up.

When we look out of our living room window, we don't see anything but trees. The trees are nice, but they are so thick that we don't even see squirrels or birds in them. There are many smaller trees that only have branches on one side of them. They can't grow because they don't get any sunlight. I want to thin them out so we can get some sunshine.

I was thinking about Kevin. I feel that he's trapped in the house. He doesn't have energy to do much, so he watches TV, which is enjoyable for him. As long as he is more comfortable on his couch, wouldn't it be nice if he could at least look outside and see birds, squirrels, and flowers? This is my new goal for now.

The weather is unusually nice, and I have decided to get going on this project. This will give Kevin a break from me hovering over him and also give me some much-needed alone time.

I was visiting with Tony and Stephanie last night. I don't know how we got on this subject but we were talking about God. I had asked them if they hear God talk to them. Stephanie told me that God talks to her a lot. She had asked me if he talks to me a lot too. I told her that I communicate with him quite often. I also told her that at times, I don't shut my mouth long enough to listen to his answer or anything he has to say either. I know I don't take the time I need with God, and I need to work on that.

Take care and have a great day!

WEDNESDAY, MARCH 17

We have been scheduled to go back to the doctor at the Mayo Clinic on April 16th for a checkup. On this appointment, they will find out how the cancer is reacting to the cancer medicines that Kevin has been taking. If the cancer cells are decreasing, Kevin will continue on the same medications. If they are not responding, the doctors will inform us of what they want to do differently.

The doctor told me that everybody reacts differently when it comes to the side effects of medicines. When side effects are listed on any medicine, they have to list *everything*. That doesn't mean that a lot of people react like this but that someone has.

I was told to call back tomorrow to see if the genetic test results were in.

THURSDAY, MARCH 18

Good news! Dr. Russell called me back and visited with me. He has a British accent, and I could listen to him talk all night long. He apologized for taking so long to get back to me but reported that the results look to be showing that Kevin is in the *standard* risk category for cancer. Kevin will need to continue the current treatment schedule. Wonderful news!

I asked Kevin if he was relieved from the test results that we were given. He replied with "I wasn't really thinking about it." Wow! I was!

Well, we have the cancer answers that we were waiting for. Now is the time to put up a good fight. Kevin has such a wonderful attitude and just continues to say, "It is what it is."

Kevin has been very stiff and sore on his chest yet. This has now spread to his back and heels too for all of this week. Remember that it was just three days ago that we were at the emergency room complaining of chest tightness.

Today, I am going to North Dakota State University for a college tour for Tony with our friends, Chris and Judy. Our boys, Ben and Tony, plan on attending college there this fall. Kevin won't be able to come with us because he will not be able to handle all of the walking.

Kevin has been driving the truck a little bit here and there, and he feels capable of driving to the doctor's office alone today in my absence. He is going to do his weekly blood draw at Buffalo, and they will again fax results to the Mayo Clinic. Kevin also will need to take his dexamethasone pills today. These really make him stir crazy, antsy, and definitely not tired. Not a good feeling to have when you're not in a situation that you can control like a college visit.

Kevin, the kids, and I are trying to schedule so many things to fit into our lives before we head down to the Mayo for the stem cell transplant. We still haven't been notified of the date that we need to be in Rochester but have an idea that it will be sometime this summer. We have graduation for Tony, confirmation for Tony and Kaylee, raising and selling chickens, getting college registration done so it's set up to move Tony to college, family pictures, doing many family activities, landscaping, and putting in the garden. Like most people, I need a plan and a schedule to go by. When this is completed, I can tackle just about anything I put my mind to.

Because of the unusually nice warm weather, the snow has melted. I have now succeeded in clearing the leaves in the grove that were packed about two and a half feet high. Now that I could see what I had to work with for clearing the grove, I started pulling all of the tiny trees out by hand. There are still a number of small, regular, and really large trees that need to be removed yet. I don't know which ones to pull so I called our friend Fred. Being as he used to do landscaping, I asked him to come over and mark the trees for me that should come down. He told me that all of the trees four-inch round or less should come down, and he marked the rest. I was all on that. I had so much fun pulling trees!

I took a log chain, put it around the trees, and pulled them out with the skid loader. I couldn't believe how many trees there were. Once they were pulled out, I piled them up and moved them to the riding arena to burn when the weather permitted. All went well, until I bent the quick-tach frame on the skid loader. I had tried to pull out a tree that was too big. I didn't do any big damage, just bent the frame, so I still could continue to work.

When Fred was over to look things over, he told me that a couple of these larger trees were too old. If they would happen to come down during a storm or anything, they could cause some serious damage to the house. He had reminded me that our friend Richard climbed trees and could possibly do this for us. I called him and he told me when he could come and take a look at the area.

We, like everyone, have family conflicts from time to time. I would like to do my best to make this home a happy home and make less conflict if I can. I realized how much easier it is to bounce the little things off in life now that normally would have bothered me in the past. When you are in a situation like this, those little things just don't seem as important after all. Now, why do we need to wait for something bigger to come along in order to deal with the little ones?

Because of this awakening that I have at the moment, I have had a chance to realize some things about myself that I don't especially care for. I tend to interrupt people when they talk and don't listen to them like I should; I don't sit with my husband at night because I see too many things that I need to do around the house; I nag at the kids about too many little things that really doesn't matter; I don't let them make their own mistakes; etc.

One day, Kevin said, "Boy, Karen, I don't know how you're going to remember all of the things that you want to change about yourself. There are so many!" We just laughed, and I called him an ass!

I don't know how Kevin will feel in the months to come, but we need to keep living, laughing, and take each day at a time. We should have been doing that already before we found out he had cancer! Thank God for another chance!

Right now, I'm feeling that my thoughts are all over the place. My mind is always racing. I ask God to use my fingers when I do these e-mails in hopes to help you all understand what is happening.

Thank you for all of the support you have shown us.

Saturday, March 20

Kevin wasn't in as much pain today. When I asked him if he is hurting, he just says, "Not really." I translate that into that he just aches. His actions look like he might have flulike aches over his whole body. I think it *really* bothers him that he hasn't been able to be at work. He must be getting sick of my smothering him and tells me at times that Kaylee and I watch him like a hawk and he can't do anything! I imagine that he must feel trapped in his own house.

Hopefully, this week he can go to work for a couple of hours a day. I think this will help his spirits and give him a better sense of normality. We will need to take one day at a time and hope that he can handle this.

Richard, who owns a local landscape business in Waverly, came over today to assess the area I have been working on. He agreed with Fred that there were trees that definitely should be cut down and that he would do it for us. I was afraid to ask how much it would cost. I knew it would be expensive but not as expensive as damage to our house.

When I read the following sentence in an e-mail that was sent to me, I thought of EACH and EVERY ONE OF YOU.

Friends are angels who lift us to our feet when our wings have trouble remembering how to fly!!"

Thank you for being my friends. I truly am blessed by God for all of you!

Tuesday, March 23

Richard came to cut down some trees today. He came with help. Oh, my! What a sight! I had no idea this was going to happen! You should have been here when the trucks came. They all had saws, ladders, oil, gas, and ropes. Our friend, Dale, and his son, Joe; Fred's son, Jacob; friend Joel; and Richard were quite the team. They were able to use our skid loader in a distance by tying one of the larger trees to it to keep it from falling toward the house when it was being cut. Not only did they cut down the larger trees, but they also cut them up for me. How wonderful! What a help! Now I can continue on my goal of opening up this area so we can use it.

I was so excited and overwhelmed with the kindness! None of the men would let me pay them for this! Richard does this for a business, and he wouldn't accept any money at all from us. The only thing they accepted was a meal. We were so grateful for their generosity. I have never experienced help from others like I have already this year. I am truly humbled.

Some of the larger trees that were cut down were too big to cut up. They needed to be split instead. I'm not familiar with using the log splitter; Kevin can't help, and I shouldn't do it alone. My sister, Penny, and her husband, Alan, told me that they would come out and help split the big logs for us. My family is amazing!

WEDNESDAY, APRIL 14

It's been a while since I last sent any updates on Kevin. He has been feeling pretty much the same as when I last updated you all. He has been going into work an average of three days a week.

Today, Kevin met with his surgeon, Dr. Garner, for a checkup on how he is healing from the neck surgery. We were told that Kevin's neck is healing well but needs to be seen again before any cell harvest and transplant for another CT scan. He wants to make sure that the tumor on his neck is gone from the radiation treatments that he has had.

Kevin was given an increase on his lifting limit to forty pounds which he really liked. The news that he *really* liked was the approval to drive his tractor and mow the lawn. The doctor also told him that he could ride in a boat as long as the water isn't wavy and choppy.

Have a wonderful day and thank you for your prayers.

THURSDAY, APRIL 15, 8:17 A.M.

I hope this doesn't make you think I am way out there with my faith, but this is what it is for me.

The news of a CT scan to verify that the tumor is gone brought me back to reality.

Kevin has been complaining every once in awhile that the left side of his neck hurts. I have been hoping and praying that this is only muscle pain. Is this the start of another race of emotions and questions? I know Kevin is in the best care with the doctors and God is on his side. I should be thinking of getting closer to the surgery and Kevin feeling better in about six months.

I prayed this morning, asking God if Kevin had a tumor on his neck again or still. I asked him to remove it if there was because we don't want another surgery. God told me, "Child of so little faith." I said in prayer, "Whatever it is, I will accept. Just please tell me." In the Bible, it says, "His will be done," and again I asked for an answer to my question. The only answer I received was that my tongue just felt swollen. I think that God was telling me not to question this. Leave it to him.

Take care and thanks for your ears.

FRIDAY, APRIL 16

It was disappointing that we still aren't scheduled for the cell harvest or bone marrow transplant yet at Rochester. We do know that it will be sometime this summer.

Today, Kevin did blood tests at the Mayo Clinic to check on the protein levels of the Myeloma cancer cells. The quantity of cancer cells that were in the marrow seem to have been reduced a lot. The doctor was very pleased with this. He had told us that the rate of cell reduction is good right now. Sometimes the number reduces quite nicely in the beginning but then the decline slows down. They will need to keep an eye on it for the next few months to be sure.

Kevin also did another skeletal infusion today, and he doesn't need to do that again for two more months or so.

While Kevin was getting his infusion, I again went to play music on the baby grand pianos at the Mayo. There are different areas around in the Mayo facilities that have piano's for others to use. I visit more than one of them so I can play the same songs over again for different groups of people. After I finished one of the songs in the large atrium, I heard someone say, "Karen, is that you?" I looked up to see if I was the Karen that this person was referring to. I couldn't believe it. I said, "Peter, is that you?" Oh my God! I haven't seen him in at least twenty-five years. We used to do quite a lot together with a fun group of people from Belle Plaine in my younger days.

Peter's girlfriend, Wendy is a friend of mine that I used to show horses with. We were both saddle club queens in the same year and had attended many of the same activities together. Peter and I visited for quite a while, and I was reminded of what a wonderful person he is. They both have already gone through more than anyone else that I have ever known in my life. They have *a lot* of health issues and go to the Mayo Clinic quite often. He reminded me that even when we are feeling down, it's good to cry. He also told me that it is a wonderful feeling and pick-me-up when you are able to help others in need. We all need to be reminded of this from time to time. Don't keep to yourself; look up and notice what else is out there for us to do in God's name.

Our next visit at the Mayo Clinic is June 8. I probably won't do Kevin updates until then, unless something unexpected comes up. Kevin will continue to get his blood and Coumadin checked in Buffalo with the results being faxed to the Mayo.

My goals to get completed before Kevin's stem cell transplant are to finish clearing out more trees on the west side of our house so Kevin can see some wildlife; do family pictures; do more things together; have Tony and Kaylee both get confirmed; Tony's graduation party; landscaping; fixing the deck and porch so Kevin has a nice place to sit and relax; pick a college registration date for Tony; and chicken orders and selling them.

We are both very tired but have the best friends anyone could ever ask for that help us and pray for us always.

FRIDAY, MAY 6, 2010

I have been the coordinator for the Howard Lake-Waverly-Winsted High School prom for two years now. It has been my responsibility to work with the students, the school, and other parents and committees to make this event a success. This was a big job. Fundraising for this year's prom started one and a half years ago. For each fundraiser, I needed to contact students and at times parental supervisors to fill the shifts. I enjoyed keeping records, organizing details for future years, and keeping a paper trail at home and at the school. I was also in charge of doing proper procedure of incoming and outgoing money and keeping records on all of it.

It's been tougher for me to do this job since we found out that Kevin has cancer. I have been trying to spend my time taking care of him and the kids. Nobody really can understand the hours that are spent calling for workers unless they have had to do it themselves at one time or another. People are either really busy, sick, out of town, or just don't want to work. I know that this will be my last year because of the unknown future of Kevin's health. I'm sad about that because I've really enjoyed getting to know and work with the kids. I really enjoy watching them grow in leadership and see the look of satisfaction on their faces when they have completed something.

We raised money all year long so kids could afford to attend this big event. We wanted each prom ticket to be as inexpensive as can be so more kids could go. The ticket price included the meal, the transportation, and the entertainment. The students did various projects to earn money instead of selling stuff. I was fortunate to usually find one or two parents who could supervise a couple of these events with me. We bagged groceries, did community paper recycling, ran concession stands at the ballpark, did car washes, etc.

I was needed at the school all day today to get the grand march list finalized, get students together for decorating the gym, help them decide how they want to decorate, and get the bus transportation lists posted.

This is such a fun time right now. The kids are pumped, and the wonderful ideas that they have for decorating is exciting.

Kevin has been a huge support for me.

SATURDAY, MAY 7

Today was the big day. It was all coming together. Girls were getting all primped up. Guys were getting their tuxedos and corsages for their dates.

It was important for me that Kevin was a part of prom this year. It's Kaylee's first prom and Tony's last. Kaylee was able to get pictures with Kevin and her uncle, Wally, this morning before she left.

Being as this is Tony's senior year, I wanted to make this special for him. I agreed that a large group of his friends could come over here for a few hours before the grand march for pictures and snacks. Our newly remodeled deck and landscaping were perfect for the backdrops.

Everything worked out so nice today. Thank you to everyone!

Chapter 8

MISHAPS AND PREPARATIONS

MAY 17, 2010, 12:41 P.M.

The last two months have been entertaining, sad, joyful, irritating, and enlightening. The following update is just a list of some of the events and mishaps that took place during this time.

It started out that I fell again at the end of March while I was working in the grove of trees. I already have TBI and am in danger of either instant death or a severe injury if I hit my head just right. This isn't a good thing for me to do. I was blessed with only receiving another small concussion and injuring my inner ear. This resulted in severe headaches and dizziness lasting continuously for a couple of weeks.

Not only did I continue to work through the pain and dizziness, but also I was bouncing in the skid loader. Working around the farm didn't help matters at all. I did too much and am thankful that the *timing was perfect*. When I could do no more, Kevin felt good enough to take care of me for a couple of weeks. I was able to get outside and work again soon but need to be aware of my surroundings and slow down this time.

This summer, I got the skid loader buried in the field. I had the forks on the front of the skid loader and not the bucket. I had no leverage, so I couldn't get myself unstuck. I ran home and told the kids that I needed them to pull me out with the truck. I tried to sneak it by without Kevin knowing because I didn't want to stress him out. We succeeded in getting that truck stuck too. Then we came home, and I had to tell Kevin what had happened. He got upset and decided that Tony, Kaylee, and he were going to get the loader unstuck and that I needed to stay home.

They came back with both trucks but no loader. All of them were mad at me again. They all couldn't believe that I got stuck! Kevin said, "Why were you there anyway? What were you thinking?" I told them that I wanted the big rock that was there. I needed it to put in my new landscaping that I'm doing. I really had no idea that it was that wet there.

Once again, I had to call on our friend, Greg. He came with his tractor the next day and pulled it out for me. When I showed him the rock that I had wanted, he laughed at me. He said that I would never have gotten that rock out. It was way too big for my equipment to handle.

Two days later, I put gas in the tractor and drove it up to a different shed. It sounded really bad, and I didn't know why. I figured that it maybe was hot or something so I shut it off and did some other work. The next day, I asked Kevin to come out and show me how to put the mower deck back on the tractor. I had told him that it wasn't running very well. I started it for him so he could hear it. I saw his face get very concerned and upset. He knows me really well and instantly asked if I put gas in instead of diesel. Boy, was this an intense moment that I thought would never end. I felt so terrible and stupid.

Thank God for good friends like Greg. He came once again to my rescue! He drained the gas line and cleaned the plugs for us. He spent a couple of hours again helping me. He made sure the tractor ran good after this was completed and checked to see if I did any damage to anything. I realize how fortunate we are to have such caring friends. The timing again was perfect because this time of year wasn't Greg's busy time yet, and he was able to squeeze this large task in.

You would think that I never ran any type of equipment before. I *always* run them! I grew up on a farm and do most of the farm stuff around here.

My *horse* died last Wednesday. As I was mowing the fence line at 6:00 a.m., I noticed that my horse was acting strange in her dry lot. She would roll, get up, run to the barn, and paw at the ground. These are signs of colic. I couldn't understand how this could be. There was no way she could have gotten into any extra feed to cause colic because I separate the horses for feeding. She was fine last night when I did chores. They have been out to pasture for some time now, and I thought that I had been monitoring the richness of the grass pretty good. I thought that maybe she was acting like this because she was hungry or bored. I decided to watch her actions some more before I did anything.

Things continued, so I called my sister, Vicki, and my veterinarian, Wes. Vicki used to have a stable and was very knowledgeable about horses and sickness. I have always relied on her wisdom about horses. My vet was busy on calls that day and lives quite a ways away from me. He agreed with what Vicki had recommended, I do to help my mare.

I tried everything I could. I walked her around for quite a while. It was cold outside, and she didn't have a problem walking but I knew that she needed a bowl movement to prove that her stomach was not twisted. Vicki suggested that I put her in the horse trailer to get her to poop. I did exactly that, and she expelled a small amount. I thought that she was okay after this, so I put her back in the dry lot. She started to eat hay, so I felt pretty good about her at the time. I checked on her from time to time.

One of the times that I came out, I noticed that she was lying down. I had a hard time getting her up, but when I did, I walked her some more. At this time, I felt helpless and didn't know what else to do. I drove her to Wes's house in Loretto. When I arrived, he gave her medicine to relax her. He was hoping that her muscles would relax and her stomach would be relieved and untwist. He tested her and said, "Some people can be sick but are strong and don't show it. Well, Cinnimon is like that. She's really a sick girl. Her internal organs are already shutting down. Because of that, my guess is that her stomach had already twisted before I spotted her at 6:00 a.m. There really isn't anything anyone can do once the stomach starts to twist."

He told me that he thought that she would make it back home in the trailer. He also told me that I did my best and I shouldn't feel bad. She was a nice horse, and I gave her a good life.

During the day and on the way home from the vet, I couldn't do anything but cry and feel like I could have done more for her. Why didn't I walk her all day? Was it too cold and because I just didn't want to? How could I do this to her? I felt terrible! Why my horse? Why not the old one?

When I arrived back home with her, I put her back in the dry lot. I thought she would at least make it to the morning. It was necessary that Kevin and I go to St. Cloud that night to get something. I explained everything in detail to the kids and reassured them that I thought she would be okay for the short time that I would be gone. I asked the kids to check on her from time to time.

We just arrived at Sam's Club and I received a panic-stricken call from Kaylee. It was terrible! My horse had been struggling so much. Kaylee's voice was in a panic as she told me what was happening! She had never experienced anything like this before. She was devastated! I'm so glad her boyfriend was with her during this time. I had to call someone to put her out of her misery right away. This was so sad and hard for me to do, but I loved her enough to let her go.

I asked Tony and Kaylee's boyfriend, Alex, to help drag her out of the dry lot and cover her up for me. Tony had never experienced handling a dead animal before. I'm sure he was scared, grossed out, and wishing he wouldn't have been home at this time. All I know is that when we came home, he looked at me with a sick look on his face and said, "I don't want to talk about it." I felt terrible that they needed to deal with this and I wasn't there. It was too late at night to do anything else but to cover her up until morning.

When I got home, I had called the rendering truck company and asked for them to pick her up. Their instructions were to leave $100 in a jar by the body for payment for their service. They would come and get her whenever they were in the area. I asked the estimated day they could come. They didn't know and guessed that they would be here sometime that week.

There is no way that I could let her lay in our yard for a week and keep a jar of money by her. Come on! I can't do that! How could I keep the wild animals away from her? I didn't want the kids to be reminded of the horror that they went through with her. How can I look at her each time I'm outside? I had no choice! Kevin and I picked a perfect spot for her grave. It is in the pasture where she always liked to be. There was an incline in the ground that I could dig into for a grave. I called our friend and asked if he could come out in the morning to haul her to the grave for me. I can do a lot of things, but I just couldn't handle finishing the job. This was so tragic for me. I got up at 5:30 a.m. and started digging a hole with the skid loader. I remember that the ground was still hard to dig into at first. Once I got started, it got easier. I managed to dig for her a hole eight to ten feet deep and wide.

As she was being taken away, my friend told me to go into the house and he would finish for me. I didn't want to do that, so I went into the barn instead and did some cleaning. When I knew he was out of sight, I went outside and cleaned up the spot that she laid. I needed this all done so after this day, it would be easier to remember how it was with her and not about what I had to clean up yet and what had happened. It was time to go forward. God blessed me with fourteen years of happiness and enjoyment with this wonderful horse. We had a lot of fun together and memories that will never go away. I gave her a good home and a great life.

Within a couple of hours one morning this last month, I assisted my chickens in murdering one of their own. The chickens were only about three weeks old at the time, so they were only about three pounds by then. In the morning, when I went to feed them, they were always so hungry. Whenever they heard my voice, they knew that food was coming and what a racket they made. As I was putting food in the pen, they all came like they were nuts. I accidentally set a feeder on one of the chickens, and I didn't know it. The other chickens trampled it. I didn't hear any struggle or peeping. As soon as I noticed one was down, it was too late. I tried to revive it by rubbing it and talking to it, but the head just dangled. I was so sad and disappointed.

I also, again, dinged the side of the shed with the corner of the tractor bucket, but thank God that it didn't break more than the metal. Good thing it was the tractor and not the skid loader. When the skid loader hits anything, it does more damage because of the power behind it.

I forgot that I was mowing the lawn with the tractor and not with the lawn mower one day. I hit the guide wire of the telephone pole with the roll bar of the tractor. Because of this, I ended up breaking the yellow protector guide on the wire. I'm thankful to have a friend that works for the power company. Chad brought out a new protector and replaced it for me.

Whenever something would go wrong, this is what happened. I would get into the house and tell Kevin, "You'll never guess what happened." He always said, "Now what did you do?" Funny, he never really seemed surprised. Can you imagine that?

I'm sure there was more that had happened, but I think you get the drift. I'm sure the tragedies that we have experienced and Karen's disaster trail are not done yet. I know, however, that with God's help, family, and community, we will get through everything. Now I'm going to list a few blessings that were given to us during the summer. This made such a huge impact on everyone involved.

As we get older, we all hope that we will be closer to our dreams and goals. Kevin and I have only been married and lived at our current home for eleven years this coming Saturday. When we moved to our home, we had dreams of what we were going to make of this place. My goal is to achieve as many of them as possible for Kevin. I want him to be relaxed and not worry about us. I want him to enjoy what he has before it's too late. I know that sounds terrible, but who knows?

Why is it that we wait until a loved one is sick to realize that our time *might* be limited to reach our goals and enjoy them? Why is it that we decide to visit with God when we are distressed and not very often when things are going our way? Why is it that we aren't happy with the things and people in our lives that God has given to us? Why do we always think the grass is greener on the other side?

We have been so very blessed with friends and family to help us achieve what I wanted to accomplish.

Kevin's brothers Lester and Wally came over and helped Tony and me spread some of the wood chips in our newly cleared-out grove.

We have always wanted to sit on the deck or in our porch and relax. We never did it. We were always too busy working and didn't take the time. Besides, both the deck and porch were in bad shape and not usable. We never took the time to fix it. Now is the time to get on top of this. Our deck on the back of our house had holes in the floor, and it hasn't been safe to walk on anymore. I was hoping that if our deck was fixed, Kevin could sit on it and relax in the sun. Our friends caught wind of it and offered their services to us. As long as we were going to replace it, we purchased maintenance-free decking. This was the best for us at this time.

Dale, Al, John, and Paul took a whole weekend out of their busy lives and replaced our deck. Steve, Tim and Laurie also came to give assistance when they could. They worked hard, long hours and didn't stop until dark. After the deck was completed, my brother-in-law, Alan; friend, Mike; his nephew; and father-in-law rescreened our porch. It previously had holes in it from the raccoons and the paint had chipped inside and out. As long as it was getting replaced, we replaced it with tongue-and-groove strip metal siding. Tony and I cleaned out the porch and repainted it to give it a brighter look.

We needed extra parking space for the graduation party, so I decided to take down one of my bigger horse pastures. I didn't have enough animals anymore to keep the grass down anyway. My sister, Penny helped me with this project while Alan was working on the porch. We rolled all of the wire and tape to store for future use. We also pulled and collected the T-posts and put them in the shed. Her help saved me so much time and backache.

My brother, Scott, knew that I needed help with some things that Kevin and I didn't get done due to Kevin's health. He asked me to get a list together of things together that I needed to get done around the farm. Things that I can't do myself like cut wood, cut down trees, carry rocks, etc. The family would get together to come out for one day and work.

On a Saturday, fourteen family members came over to help us get things done. Alan, Jeff, and Brent cut a ton of wood for us, split it, and stacked it for winter. Alan, Gary, and Jeff installed the screen door that we had purchased four years ago for outside the laundry room. Penny, Scott, Brenda, Ryan, Jackie, Meghan, Jessica, Kaylee, Stephanie, Dad, and I did landscaping. Together we were able to create a new landscape and fix some of the existing landscape around our house. Both my mom and grandma were in wheelchairs and wanted to help. They also needed to be included in helping us with something. I remembered that I didn't have time to finish the tie blankets for Kevin and me when he was at Abbott hospital. My mom and grandma, who was ninety-six years old finished tying them to completion for us.

Our friend, Trudy, took the leftover material from the tie blankets and made Viking pillows for Kevin. Inside one of the pillows, she inserted a note of paper with a special prayer for Kevin on it. Kevin was instructed to leave it in the pillow.

I don't have a green thumb, nor was I ever interested in plants before now. My sister-in-law and friend, Jill, had given and planted some plants for us in the areas that needed it. This all was done in half of a day. When people work together and have a plan, it really doesn't take long.

My friend, Jill, came and helped me fix the edge of the center island that used to be the grove of trees. We dug up and replaced all of the rocks that were already there.

We had so much help preparing for graduation also. Our friend, Mary, came over and helped me paint the garage wall so it looked nice for graduation. Al, Dede, Sandy, Mary, Jill, and Dale came over to help us clean out the big shed for graduation so if it rained, we could move the party to the shed.

I had visited with Karen, our youth director at church, previously about taking our family pictures. I wanted them done before we went to Rochester for the transplant. You never know what will happen down there. Sad to say but what if Kevin doesn't come back home? We need to have a family picture for memories. The picture on the cover of the book was taken at this time.

I have a huge garden each year that is 150 feet long by 50 feet deep. Each year, I fill the garden with tomatoes, beans, cucumbers, corn, potatoes, and other miscellaneous vegetables. This spring, I had already decided to plant my garden this year and share the fruit it produced with friends and family. This is something that I can do for them.

Take care and *make* today a great day! I love all of you and am grateful to God that you are a part of our lives.

THURSDAY, JUNE 3, 2010

Kevin went to see his surgeon who fused his neck. Dr. Garner told us that the neck is healing well and told Kevin that he can expect to have pain for a while yet. Kevin will not have any other appointments with this doctor anymore, unless his neck pain gets worse.

SUNDAY, JUNE 6

Tony and Kaylee were confirmed today. They both gave powerful testimonies of their faith in front of the congregation. Family, friends, and church members were all touched by the messages that the kids had shared.

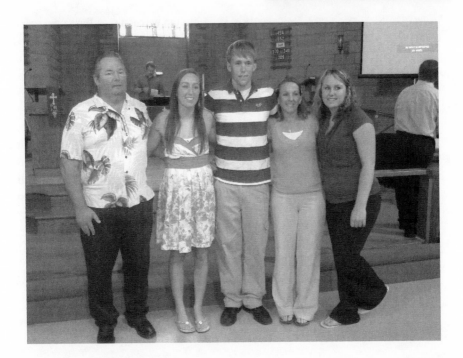

Wow! They grew up! I felt truly blessed and thankful of the faith they have in our Lord Jesus Christ. I felt comforted that Tony and Kaylee know that they can rely on God to carry them when they need support. I felt that they have experienced a relationship with God and will keep him close.

After church service, we took pictures with the kids and then went to the narthex for coffee hour to visit with others. The church board always supplies a confirmation cake for this celebration for everyone to enjoy. This was a very emotional celebration that was amazing in itself.

We invited our immediate family, the church youth director and her family to come to our home to have lunch afterwards. Shortly after the meal, it was time for everyone to change clothes. It was high school graduation time for Tony.

The graduation ceremony was at the high school. Most of the family stayed to celebrate the ceremony with us and take more pictures. Tony now will be starting his new chapter in his life and we are so proud of him.

It was an amazing day! We succeeded in separating the celebrations and keeping them each as special as they could be.

Tuesday, June 8, 2010

We went down to the Mayo for another skeletal infusion. Kevin also had some blood tests to track how the cancer cells are reacting to the medicines. Results showed the cancer cells are continuing to die. This is good! They are dying at a slower pace, but that was expected. Everything seems to be going the way it needs for Kevin to get healthy again. The bone marrow transplant and all of the other pretransplant work will be started July 6th at the Mayo. We will be staying down there for six to eight weeks.

Kevin needs a caretaker with him 24/7, so we are planning on having replacements from time to time so I can come home and support the kids and relieve them from the daily chores.

Kevin and I were able to take a tour of the Gift of Life Transplant House. We toured the oldest one of the two houses. These houses are for transplant patients and their caretakers to stay at during their medical visits at the Mayo Clinic.

The house that we visited has forty-eight rooms for patients and is usually full. It's not home, but it will be just right for the time being. This is where we want to stay during our time in Rochester because it's affordable, and it will be the most sanitary place available for us. We are hoping that they have an empty room for us on July 6. They will call us a couple days in advance to confirm with us whether they have a room for us or not. If they don't, we will need to stay elsewhere until a room opens up.

Thank you for all of your prayers. I will e-mail when we are down at the Mayo Clinic and have new news to share. God bless you and yours!

TUESDAY, JUNE 15, 2010

We planned on having our family pictures taken today. It is sad, but you know when you go to funerals, you see all the pictures of memories that were shared. Well, I don't feel that I have taken enough pictures throughout our life together. We don't know for sure if Kevin will come back after Rochester or how his health will be or how he will look either. We want to have a family picture to capture us together before the Rochester visit. We also want current pictures to look at while we are away from each other.

It was terribly difficult for Kevin to do this. He was very weak, sore, and tired. He felt the same way and knew how important this was. He told me while the pictures were being taken, "I hope this is over soon. I don't know how much more I can take." Well, he managed to struggle through.

Karen was wonderful, understanding, quick and still managed to take a couple hundred pictures. After these pictures were taken, Kevin went back to work. Karen had suggested going back to our home so she could take some group pictures of the kids and also individual pictures of each child.

Tony didn't appreciate this as much as the girls, but went along with it for a little while anyway. The girls felt so special and really loved that one on one picture time. Karen was really creative and took pictures of the kids in the field, smelling flowers, by the house, you name it. This was so appreciative and wonderful.

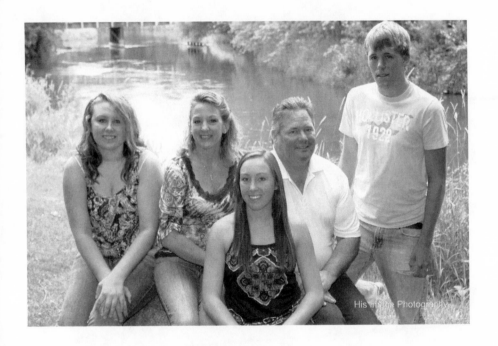

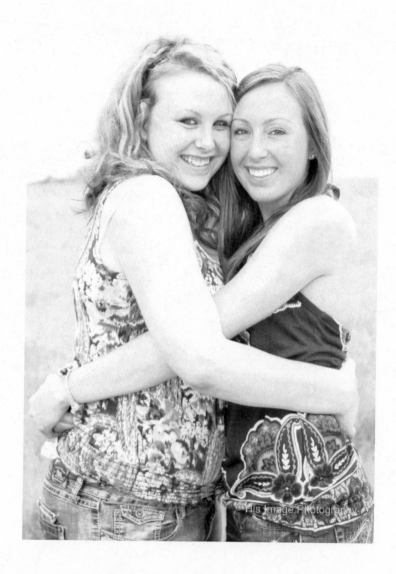

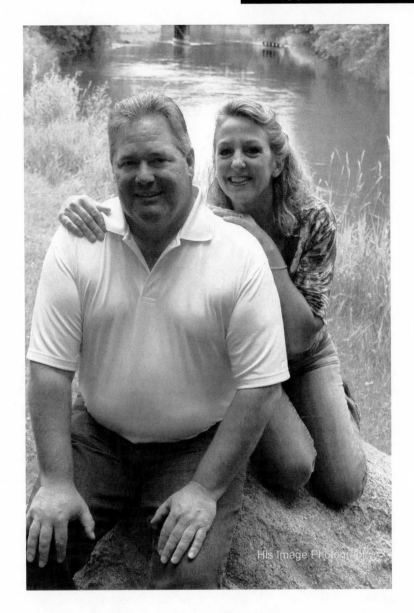

JUNE 19, 2010

We had Tony's graduation party today. Our home looked magnificent, thanks to the help of so many friends and family. We had a feast of food and drink.

We invited all of Kevin's relation that he hasn't seen in many years. We wanted to reconnect with all of them before heading to the Mayo Clinic.

It was truly a long day for Kevin, and he was exhausted. We had so much fun, and it was a wonderful day and celebration.

FRIDAY, JULY 2, 2010

We were told that they had a room for us at the Gift of Life House. This is what we were hoping for. They said that we can stay there for the entire time that we are down there for treatment. The cost savings alone was a blessing and necessity.

We were accepted into the newer of the two Gift houses. We haven't seen this one but heard that it's really nice. Now that we know where we are going to stay, we have a better idea of what items we need to pack. I'm not very excited about sharing a house with other people. I have never been in this kind of living situation before. I'm nervous and thinking the worse. I know this is wrong, but I don't want to get let down.

MONDAY, JULY 3, 2010

How do we prepare for this trip to Rochester? I was already heartbroken just thinking of being away from the kids. What else could I do? I was reminded that the Gift of Life House told us that Kevin would need a caretaker twenty-four hours a day and seven days a week. He was not to be left alone at all! Remember when I told you that I would get relief caretakers from friends and family so I could come home from time to time? Well, there are so many important rules to follow at the Gift House that we both felt that it would be almost impossible for me to come home at all during his entire stay. If somebody new would come to be with him, they wouldn't know what was needed. It would be too difficult.

We were told that the approximate amount of time for our stay in Rochester would be four to six weeks. We were hoping that this time would go by faster than we could imagine so we just asked some people to check on things at home from time to time. Thank God for phones, which will give us an opportunity to hear the kids' voices and communicate with them personally. This will be a big help for all of us. The three kids already had to be alone for the most part while Kevin and I were at Abbott NW Hospital in December and January.

I had written earlier about the phone call I received in January from Tony. The girls were fighting, and he didn't know what to do. All I could hear in the background was screaming and crying. They had reached their max and needed parental support. Because of this, we felt that our decision of separation for the kids would be healthier for each one of them. If all of the kids would be home together with no parental supervision, it would be nothing but trouble. They will fight and try to pass work on to the youngest one as often as they could.

We had made arrangements for Stephanie to live with her father in Minnetonka, while Kevin and I were gone. She seemed sad about this, and I could tell there was some concern as to if she'd miss her friends and home. Deep down, she knew that this would be the best thing to do. She loves her dad and has wanted to have more time with him in the past anyway, so this is her chance.

I was really sad that the siblings would be forty-five minutes apart. I know that they love and need each other. I felt comforted that they could call each other if anything was needed or just wanted to talk. Stephanie will miss her friends. Her father and we assured her that she could come back home a few times to get together with them. We felt bad that she needed to pack up and leave her normal life here but felt that we really didn't have any choice in the matter.

I felt comfortable with all of our planning. We have scheduled people to look in on Tony and Kaylee from time to time. We have great neighbors that can keep watch on the farm also in our absence.

We still have our list of names and phone numbers of people who have offered help and support this past December and January. The kids would be able to call anyone when they ever need anything. I instructed Tony and Kaylee how to sort and wash clothes. Tony is familiar with the skid loader and tractor, so if anything needed to be done, he can do it alone. He was put in charge of horse chores and mowing the grass. He also was aware that the garden needed to be watered from time to time and assured me that he would tend to this too.

I asked Kaylee to keep the garden free from weeds. I also instructed her as to how and how often to spray the weeds in the center island and landscape around the house. She also was to feed the dogs. The kids were to keep the house in order and have no parties. They were to make sure that one of the two of them was at home most of the time and every night. The dogs will miss me, and they need to be kept as normal as possible too.

Sunday, July 4, 2010

Paul and Rita had their annual Fourth of July party on the lake. It's like a community celebration. This was an opportunity for Kevin and me to see some of our friends before the journey to Rochester. It was comforting to hear them all tell us that they will continue their prayers for healing.

Chapter 9

MAYO CLINIC

MONDAY, JULY 5, 2010

Today is the day. I was distressed and sad to leave the kids and the farm. We were both filled with so many emotions. We were happy that the day finally came. It seems like we have been waiting for this step in Kevin's healing for a long time.

We were hopeful and counting on a short stay in Rochester and reminded ourselves that the time would fly by quicker than we could imagine and we'd be home in no time.

Kevin and I arrived at Rochester around nine thirty tonight. We want to settle in, and I will e-mail again tomorrow.

TUESDAY, JULY 6, 2010, FIRST E-MAIL
(UPDATE TYPED WEDNESDAY, JULY 7, 4:30 P.M.)

A little history on the Gift of Life Houses.

Edward Pompeian, a Mayo Clinic kidney transplant patient, was instrumental in developing the first transplant house in 1973. His own experience with the needs of transplant patients and their families led him to believe that a shared environment in a home setting would be beneficial to all concerned.

There are currently two Gift of Life Houses in Rochester, which accommodates a total of eighty-seven guest rooms between them. We have a private bedroom with two double beds and a bathroom with a walk-in shower. I was so relieved the second we stepped into our room. We are blessed to have a corner room. It seems to be much bigger than what we had seen in the old house.

We have our own small dry storage place by the kitchen, our own shelf in the refrigerator, and a basket in the freezer to store our frozen foods. We share the rest of the house with the other patients, their caretakers, and the visiting guests. We have access to the kitchen, dining room, patio, and grill; a choice of various TV rooms; an exercise room; a library; a coin laundry room; a computer room; and quiet rooms. There are also games, a piano, a sewing machine, and puzzles to occupy your time and mind.

There are also activities planned at times for everyone in hopes of getting people out of their rooms and to socialize. They make it as comfortable as they can for us here. They really understand how difficult it is to be away from home and your loved ones.

There are *a lot* of rules that go along with being able to stay here. It's very important to keep all illnesses away due to the health and immune systems of the guests. Disinfect, disinfect, disinfect. I am *not* a very ambitious cleaner. I am good at picking up but not disinfecting.

I also believe that by being here, the healing and comfort is going to be *much* better than if Kevin had to stay in the hospital.

Kevin is exhausted right now but is very comfortable at the moment. We have had a very full day of appointments that went from 7:00 a.m. to 4:30 p.m. Kevin called the nurses vampires because of all the blood that they needed to take. He got poked and prodded a lot today and has kept track of how many vials of blood they took from him. His comment is "I don't think I have much blood left in me."

We were given a *ton* of information at each appointment today about the procedures ahead of us. We were overwhelmed at times but tried to focus and understand what was being explained to us. I will give details tomorrow because I'm pooped out right now and my brain isn't working anymore.

Kevin and I are so very thankful for the prayers and the support you all have given us!

Oh, by the way, Monday night, the first thing Kevin and I both needed to do was read the manual for explaining all of the rules of the house. We needed to sign forms saying that we read and understand them all. Well, this morning, Kevin told me that he read in the manual that I can't nag at him for anything while we stay at the Gift of Life House. He just doesn't quit. He always makes me laugh and brightens my day. I love him so much! Kevin's spirits are great!

I will keep in touch. God bless!

TUESDAY, JULY 6, 2010, DAY 1, SECOND E-MAIL
(UPDATE ALSO TYPED WEDNESDAY, JULY 7, 4:30 P.M.)

This was our first day of screening appointments at the Mayo Clinic. The screening tests are done to determine if Kevin's health will allow him to have the transplant, identify problems that may affect the transplant process, and document the current status of his cancer. These tests included evaluation of the function of his vital organs, tests to screen for infections, x-rays, and scans. They communicated the necessary details of these procedures to us.

We had meetings with the transplant coordinator and the division of hematology first. They discussed some studies that they are conducting at the Mayo Clinic with us. These studies are done in hopes of improving the treatment of this disease in the future. They felt that Kevin was an ideal candidate to participate in these tests because of his age and health. We were given all of the facts necessary for us to decide if we will or will not participate. Kevin agreed to be a part of these tests. We feel that medicine has come a long way due to the studies like these in the past.

Kevin needed to fill out some forms, answering questions about his lifestyle, how he feels right now, and other miscellaneous things. He will need to repeat these questions again next year for the transplant study for a comparison of his health and life changes. This reminded me to request the living will and advance directives form for us to fill out. This form will describe the treatment preferences we have in an end-of life situation. I also got one for myself because I thought it was necessary and would help Kevin if I also filled one out for myself.

To complete one of the tests, Kevin needed to give extra blood and extra bone marrow during his normally scheduled extraction. He will only need to do this one time for the hematology study that is being conducted. After that, Kevin went to have his bone marrow biopsy. They take a very long needle and insert it in his backside to extract bone marrow. This is done for testing and comparison to the last collection.

Later in the day, I forgot that Kevin had this test done. He had a patch above his right butt cheek where they inserted the needle. We were joking around, and I slapped him there. I got his attention for sure that time. Later, I needed to check the patch to make sure that it didn't start to bleed from my slap. I was relieved not to find blood! Isn't it fun living with me?

The next appointment for the day was blood and urine testing. Finally at 10:30 a.m., we could get coffee and something to eat.

We then had an appointment with a doctor explaining to us the intravenous catheter or sometimes called a "central line" that they will use for this transplant procedure. The catheter is a thin flexible tube that will be inserted into a large vein in his chest or neck. The catheter is used to deliver medicine, nutrition, blood transfusions, and the healthy blood stem cells. It is also used to draw blood for the frequent blood tests that Kevin will need during the transplant process. A surgeon or radiologist made two small incisions in Kevin's chest and threaded this catheter through a large vein until it approached his heart. This tube will remain in place until his treatment here in Rochester is completely finished.

We were given a tour of the cell harvest area. The medical staff explained to us the harvest process. We also were able to see the machines that would be used for collection.

Kevin had an electrical impedance cardiogram and then took two x-rays. Kevin told me that he couldn't believe how many x-rays they took. They took some, called the doctor to look, took some more, and so on. He said, "I bet they took twenty x-rays! Thank God for insurance!"

There was no time to fit in our social-worker consultation today, so it was rescheduled for tomorrow.

Being as we got in so late on Monday night, we really didn't get settled in at the house yet. We went shopping for cleaning supplies and some other necessities before heading back to the Gift of Life House.

As soon as we got home and unpacked, I looked and Kevin was sleeping. I was afraid to let him continue sleeping because it was so early in the evening. I didn't want him to wake up in the middle of the night and get his sleep pattern screwed up. I tried but wasn't able to keep him awake. He was so exhausted.

I needed to print some paperwork off and went to the computer room that the house provided. The gentleman using the computer next to me started talking about some woman getting stoned to death in Iran for adultery. I told him, "Wow! We all commit adultery at some time." Well, he told me that I didn't know what I was talking about.

After that, he was talking about the Old Testament and how the women *and* men who committed adultery were stoned. I then (not always knowing what I'm talking about) thought I'd take a stab and said, "King David didn't get stoned. He even sent the husband of who he wanted to war so he would be out of the way." This man told me! "That's not what happened. Men who went to war divorced their wives before they went to war. They did this just in case the woman found someone else and didn't want to wait for them to get back from war. It wasn't considered adultery." He said, "You just don't know." I changed the subject really fast.

Kevin, the kids, and I are all doing well! We are blessed that I can be here with Kevin during this time.

Love to each one of you!

WEDNESDAY, JULY 7, 2010, 9:20 P.M., DAY 2

Kevin had slept straight through the night. I even had to shake him to get him up at 6:00 a.m.

Today was another day of screening. They are so very professional and thorough here at the Mayo Clinic.

At 7:00 a.m., Kevin had an appointment for a pulmonary function test dilator. This was comprised of a ton of breathing tests that Kevin did to check that his lungs were functioning properly. One test was to measure the amount and rate of airflow going into and out of the lungs. Another test was to measure the maximum amount of air you could inhale and how much air your lungs contain when you have exhaled. Another test measured how well gases, such as oxygen, move from the lungs into the blood, and the pulse oximetry test measures the level of oxygen that's in your blood.

After that appointment, Kevin had an echocardiogram, which is like an ultrasound to take pictures of your heart to make sure it is functioning properly.

Then we went to an education class teaching ME how to care, clean, and change the dressing of the intravenous catheter that Kevin will have for this procedure. I was worried that I would forget what I was told and screw something up. I was also concerned that I would not clean the area good enough and he would get infection. That could be fatal for Kevin! What stress this was for me!

My headaches are still *really* bad. We have been going up and down in the elevators so much, and I have been dizzy more than usual. My inner ear still was an issue at this time yet. I have been trying to get in to see a specialist here at the Mayo for my head issues but have not had success.

We have both been overwhelmed with everything that we have been told. There were so many rules, schedules, statistics, numbers, important instructions for caring for my husband, etc. I remember leaving the room from this education class and was overcome with the feeling to just fall down and hit my head. The doctors will have to see me then. Get hurt and they will have to see you. Get another concussion and they will see you now! I didn't do it but a short while later had another bout of feelings to just fall down the stairs. The doctor's will see that they need to see me then. They won't be able to turn me down.

I couldn't believe that I got to this point. I realized that the evil one was putting these thoughts in my head. I was not going to let him do this to me! He knew I was weak and needed help, and he thought that he was going to take over. Really! How would hurting myself benefit me? What good would it do Kevin and the kids? I prayed, "In the name of Jesus, be gone!" The feeling left me. I was free to continue care for Kevin.

After the education class, we were able to make up the session that we missed yesterday with the transplant center social worker. The time given for this consultation was well worth it. When we left this meeting, we felt comfortable knowing that we had been scheduled one person to contact if we were ever confused about anything or needed anything.

We took some time to walk around and enjoy a small part of Rochester. As we were enjoying each other's company, I decided to call home and talk to the kids. I couldn't find my phone and realized that I had lost it or left it somewhere. I panicked. We stood still for a moment and retraced our steps and stops in our minds. What a relief! We realized where it was, and I told Kevin to just stay put and I will run and get it. He was really tired and pretty weak at this time. We had done a lot of walking already. I knew that going with me would be too much for him, so he found a spot to sit while I went to retrieve my phone.

On the way, I noticed an elderly woman trying to cross the street. She looked very frustrated. Because of her age and how slow she walked, the traffic signs changed before she got very far. People are so rude! Cars wouldn't wait for her. Traffic was busy at this time and I was able to help her cross safely. I remember needing to put my hand out to a car to make them stop for her. Once we had crossed the street, she extended her sincere thanks to me. She was so sweet! As I was walking away from her, she got my attention and blew me a kiss! I guess I was at the right place at the right time. She made my day today.

I finally arrived back to Kevin with my phone. I excitedly told him how I was able to help this old woman. I felt so good to do this. We decided to go back to the house for the rest of the day. We have had a very big day today already and are both exhausted.

When we got back to the house, I had learned some more information about the kitchen duties that were required of me. I had some time and met a few of the patients and caregivers that are sharing the house with us. Everyone here so far is so very friendly, kind, and helpful. I know God will use Kevin and me while we are here in some shape or form. Kevin has a great attitude and seems content as long as I am here with him. It makes me feel good when he asks where I've been or "Why are you going to read in the dining room when you can read here?" He needs me, and we are content together.

Tomorrow is a huge day for us. We have appointments from 9:15 a.m. to 4:00 p.m. and will be meeting with some doctors regarding Kevin's treatment. I am feeling strong, knowing that our kids know how to rely on Jesus for strength, and we keep in contact with them daily to give them support. I will e-mail tomorrow again!

Thursday, July 8, 2010, 6:19 p.m., day 3

We slept in today because our first appointment wasn't until 9:15 a.m. We had a very busy day with schedules and met with our coordinator and three doctors.

Good news! All of Kevin's tests came back good! Thank you, God, and thank you too for all of your prayers!

Kevin's I&R is too high; however, this can be fixed with medication. When Kevin had his blood clot in the hospital in January, they put him on Coumadin to make his blood thinner. They did this to reduce clotting of the blood. The goal since then has been to keep his blood regulated at 2.5 to 3.0 until they feel he didn't need this anymore. This means that if I would get a cut and Kevin would get a cut, it would take Kevin two and a half to three times faster to stop bleeding or clot than me. Kevin's blood needed to be thicker in order to perform the surgery for putting the catheter in place. If the blood would be thinner than 1.5, Kevin could bleed to death while they are inserting the catheter. The doctors switched the strength of his Coumadin to correct this problem.

The doctors decided to do cell collection for three transplants instead of two. One cell collection will be used now, and the other two cell collections will be frozen for use at a later date. If and when Kevin would need another transplant, he would already have clean cells to transplant. Wonderful! This means that they will be collecting twelve million stem cells instead of eight million. Isn't this amazing?

Next, the process *before* the stem cell collection is called priming. This too needs to be done before the cell collection. Kevin is getting his first shot of this tomorrow morning at 7:30 a.m. Priming is the mobilization and colony-stimulating factor of stem cells and is done by using a drug called Neupogen. Neupogen is given by injection four days prior to stem cell collection and continues until harvesting is complete. This injection will increase the number of cells that are transferred from the bone marrow into the bloodstream.

In Kevin's case, instead of using the drug Neupogen, the whole time, Kevin will switch to a test-study medicine. This is called Plerixafor, which is given by IV instead, for the remaining time of priming and during the cell harvest. The cost of this IV med is $6,000 per dose. The Mayo Clinic waives the fee for the test participants. This will save the insurance company $24,000.00 by Kevin participating in the study.

This medication stimulates the stem cells even more than the Neupogen. The reason it's not used the entire priming and collection time is because it can only be used for a total of four days.

After we got all of this information, Kevin needed to see the dentist who only does oral surgery to check and make sure he doesn't have any teeth that would fall out or cause a problem with infections at any time during or after this transplant procedure. He currently was cleared to go forward with everything.

My feelings are overwhelmed, in awe of the amazing medical technology, exhausted, happy, blessed, impressed with the professionalism of everyone we've met, glad to be here, miss home, terrible headaches, unknowing, and relieved.

We trust in God, our Lord and Savior. We have given the cancer cells to him repeatedly to do what he wants with them.

Kevin and I will continue to be strong for each other, and our family and friends, whom we *love so very much*! Thank you for your support!

Our schedule will change tomorrow a lot, so I will keep in touch with you.

Friday, July 9, 2010, 12:52 P.M., day 4

Today was pretty uneventful. Kevin had his first primer shot of Neupogen. We ended up waiting a while for the nurse, but she said that was unusual. We also had another class on the transplant procedure. I will e-mail details about that when it happens.

Kevin and I are *really pooped*! We both are doing well, and so are the kids and the home place.

Kevin will be taking another set of primer shots Saturday and Sunday in the morning. We will find out Sunday night as to how his blood thickness is doing. It's possible that we will also be able to set up the next shot appointment and the surgery date to insert the catheter.

Thank you and have a wonderful weekend.

Saturday, July 10, 2010, 9:15 a.m., day 5

We have been sleeping well and are very comfortable here.

Kevin had another primer shot treatment this morning.

We are asking everyone we know to please NOT send real plants, food, etc., or anything here for Kevin. Soon, Kevin can't be around plants. Dirt is mold and Kevin could get sick from it. Kevin also will be limited to certain food types due to impurities. Boy, oh boy, are we are learning a lot!

We also were talking and confirmed our earlier decision of nobody relieving me even for one or two days. There is so much to know and look for right now. We explained the reasons to the kids and told them that they will need to come down here every once in a while to visit us. They are welcome any time and that we are still here for them.

Kevin told me that last night he was thinking about being down here and what we have all learned. He said to me, "Karen, it takes how many days to form a habit? I think we'll be here that long and you might actually carry this cleaning thing home with us." I told him, "Very unlikely!" Ha ha ha!

Realizing that this weekend *might* be the last weekend that Kevin will feel like going out and about, we're going to visit Soldier's Field Vet Memorial in Rochester and go grocery shopping.

It is wonderful weather here, and we hope you all have a wonderful weekend. God bless!

SUNDAY, JULY 11, 2010, 3:32 P.M., DAY 6

This morning, Kevin told me that he had kind of a rough night with a little pain. This is very common in this stage of treatment. The cells are starting to multiply in his bone marrow and are causing his bones to hurt. He said that when the pain came, it was as if he could feel those little suckers, the cells, talking.

Patients who have a bone marrow graft usually have pain in the lower back where the graft was done first. Usually pain resides in the middle of the chest soon after.

Kevin's spirits are still wonderful; he had his third set of primer shots this morning and blood draw to test how his blood is.

Tonight, we can call to see what our schedule for tomorrow is.

This morning, I was watching the nurse while she was in with Kevin. She was using a bar code machine on Kevin's wristband and the bar codes on each medicine that she was going to use. This was just like in the grocery store. I was curious about it, so of course, I inquired about the procedure she was doing. Kevin has a bar code associated with his name. His medicines, doses, quantities, and any other miscellaneous things the medical staff needs to know are all programmed into the computer.

The pharmacy is notified instantly if the bar code is activated on a medicine that is different than what's on Kevin's records. It won't let the wrong bar code be accepted into the computer at the time it's scanned if it's wrong. This would then alert the nurse that she has the wrong medicine.

An example for this would be a patient on an IV infusion. The bracelet bar code gets scanned and then the IV bar code is scanned. If everything matches, the bar code charts the infusion as ordered by the medical doctor. *But* accidents do happen. Medical staff could be rushed or just not paying attention. Bar coding prevents medical errors.

What a safety feature! We were told that more and more hospitals want to go to that kind of computer system.

I went to church this morning at the Christian church across the street. There was a short story on the back of the bulletin that talked about needing a transfusion. Of course, that caught my attention! The kind of transfusion I read was of God's love. Basically it told me that true love isn't within us and true forgiveness can't be found in our hearts on our own. We can only get true love and forgiveness from an outside source. We need a transfusion of God's love and forgiveness to fill our hearts, souls, and minds. We need to be filled with the Holy Spirit. God loved us first and died on the cross to save us from our sins, even though he knew that we would continue to sin. This is agape love.

I asked God for a continued renewal of a transfusion. I am in need of true patience, kindness, peace, generosity, sympathy, calmness, and a sense of humor.

This church I attended also runs a couple of compassion houses in Rochester. These homes are rent-free for any patient who is in need of housing during their treatment. It's for patients that *do not* need disinfected kitchens, homes, or rooms.

My sister, Penny, and her husband, Alan, came down today and drove us to Lanesboro to go antiquing and a drive. We were really tired and not especially looking forward to more running but needed to be with family. Kevin's only concern about the travel plans was that he wanted to make sure that he would be able to get his piece of blueberry pie at the Lanesboro pie shop.

When we got back from Lanesboro and the pie shop, Kevin and I realized how much we really needed this trip. It was like we escaped and had fun! We were so grateful for such a wonderful day made possible only because of them. Alan and Penny sure put the miles on for us! They drove from Waconia to Rochester to Lanesboro to Rochester and back to Waconia again.

I will e-mail you all tomorrow. Take care and love life!

MONDAY, JULY 12, 2010, 9:30 P.M., DAY 7

At 7:00 a.m. this morning, Kevin and I were at the clinic for the surgical procedure of installing the intravenous catheter.

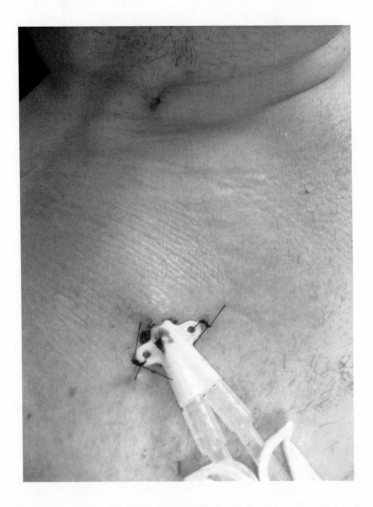

The spot up by Kevin's neck (upper left), just below his neck and jaw, is where the insert was. I don't know if you can see but the bump (or puff) is the tube under Kevin's skin. This tube goes into the main artery by the heart and out where you see the connectors are.

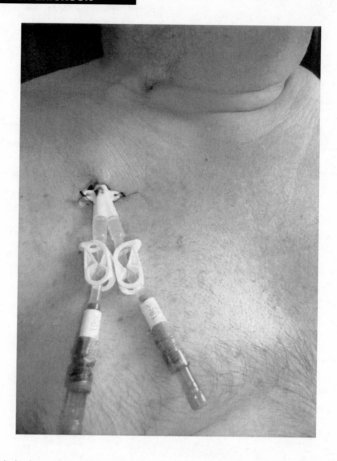

This is the catheter. It has one port for extraction of cells and one port for reinsertion of reheated cells. There are two ends to this connector. The left one, as you are looking at it, is the output, and the right side is the input. The two white things you see on each tube are clips to close or lock the tube until needed for injection, medications, etc. The green caps also seal the tubes. Each time the doctors need to do something, they remove the caps. Whenever the caps are removed, everyone needs to have masks on and the area or room needs to be disinfected. This is so no germs get into the bloodstream. The staff first sucks or pulls out the blood that was stored in the tube between the heart and the end caps. They then flush the line clean and can continue on with what they need to do.

Kevin told me about the preoperation rooms at the clinic. The preop room numbers for men starts with the letter *m* and those for women starts with *f*. The operation tags that were put on the gurney for men were blue and the women's were pink. Everywhere he went they asked him who he was, who his doctor was, and what he was having done.

Kevin received his fourth primer shot to increase cell production.

Kevin's neck doesn't move well, due to his fusion this past December. He has even less movement of his neck now because of this surgery, but it should loosen up in a few days. He doesn't have too much pain at the moment and has a *great* attitude.

We decided that I would sleep in the other bed in our room at the transplant house until this catheter was removed. Kevin needs to be comfortable, and we need to protect the catheter.

Tomorrow, we are scheduled for appointments starting at 6:30 a.m. and should be done midafternoon.

Nothing much happened here today, other than meeting a few more people at the house and getting excited for Stephanie and Kaylee to come down Wednesday afternoon for a visit.

Take care and have a great night.

TUESDAY, JULY 13, 2010, 3:27 P.M., DAY 8

Kevin didn't get much sleep last night. He was very uncomfortable due to the placement of the catheter and his stiff neck.

As I explained earlier, Kevin already received four primer shots of Neupogen. He will need to continue them during the whole collection process.

This morning, Kevin had his catheter dressing changed and his first IV of Plerixafor. Kevin is the ninth patient to ever use this drug. This medicine, as I explained earlier, is a new study for increasing cell production *above and beyond* the current medicine he is also receiving as a primer. The reason to include this medicine now is that they can only administer this for four days prior to transplant. Side effects known from this drug are bone, joint, or muscle pain; diarrhea; nausea; vomiting; dry mouth; increased sweating; headache; etc. We will need to call the doctor if he starts itching and swelling, and having tingling in his mouth, chest tightness, burning, numbness, lightheadedness, shortness of breath, unusual bleeding, fever, etc.

It's 2:00 p.m. right now, and it has been six and a half hours since he was first administered this drug. He has not shown any symptoms of the above side effects at this time.

Kevin had a shot for a blood thinner around 10:00 a.m. and needed to wait one hour or so before they could start the collection and extraction process of cells.

At the time, I'm typing this e-mail and Kevin called me on my cell phone. He told me that I'm not allowed back in the collection room. He said that I fed him the wrong breakfast this morning and the nurses are upset. He started laughing and I could hear the nurses laughing in the background too. Yes, I can go back in the area, Kevin was just teasing me. Evidently, he wasn't supposed to have scrambled eggs or sausage this morning. This causes the collection of cells to be discolored. The cells were a milky color, and they're supposed to be clear. Neither one of us remembers reading any information like this! I made sure to get a list of foods that he can and can't eat while he is in the collecting stage this week.

The nurses on that floor are wonderful, professional, and will be really fun to be around. They get a kick out of Kevin's sick sense of humor. The following is a brief description of the collection for those who are interested.

A recap. During these past months, Kevin was given medications to decrease the cancer cells in his bone marrow. This doesn't mean that the cancer cells are gone. It means that there are just not as many that are infected with the cancer disease because the medicine treated them.

The primer shots that he has already received the last four days are increasing the production of the current cells in his bone marrow. The cells are increasing so much that they have nowhere to go other than flowing over into the bloodstream. This is exactly where they want them because they will be collecting them from the blood.

Today the additional medication, Plerixafor, was administered. This will increase the production of cells even more. Remember that they want to collect twelve million of these cells.

The nurse attached the exit line from Kevin's catheter to the machine that will extract the cells. Once the cells are transferred, they will at this time be separated by the machine. The stem cells, which are the good fighting cells, will be removed or separated from the red cells and platelets. There is a spinner that you can hopefully see by the picture that does the separating. The stem cells will be saved for the transplant. The red cells and the platelets are put back into Kevin as soon as they are separated. This is done also from the machine through the entrance site of the catheter. This whole process is a continuous, slow-going process.

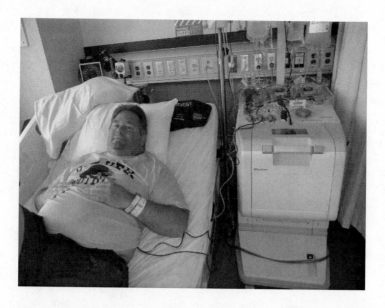

Kevin will be hooked up to this machine for up to five hours each day until enough cells are collected.

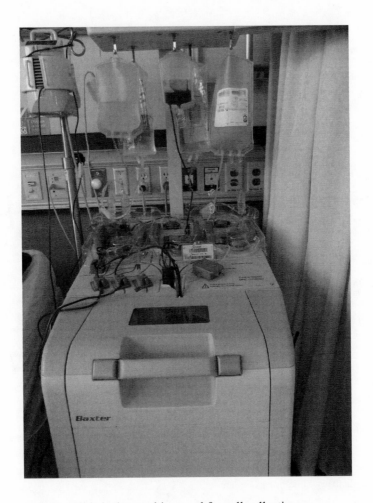

This is the machine used for cell collection.

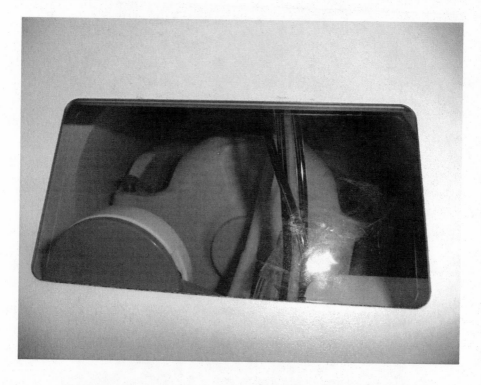

This is the drum in the machine that the extracted cells from Kevin go first. This drum spins and separates the stem cells, red cells, and platelets. The stem cells go to the top of the drum due to the cell's lighter weight. From here, they go out of the drum and into a collection bag. These are the stem cells that will be frozen for later use.

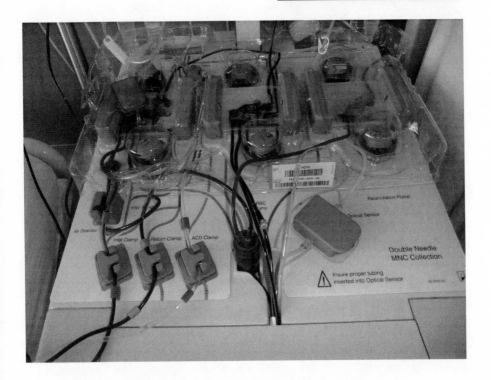

The other cells run into different bags, which will then go through a tube to get reheated so Kevin's body doesn't get cold when they are sent back through the tube to the input connection and back into Kevin's bloodstream.

Earlier I showed a picture of Kevin's catheter. One connection is used for the extraction of cells; and one connection, for input or reinsertion of cells. During the collection time, Kevin's blood temperature needs to be controlled, and a nurse is continuously watching to make sure everything is going as planned.

This will be our schedule for the rest of the week. To the hospital at 6:30 a.m. for an IV of Plerixafor, shot of primers at 9:30 a.m., and two hours later is the collection time for up to five hours. The only addition to this schedule is a class on psychiatry/psychology.

Kevin and I have an area by the window during this collection time and a television made available for us to watch. We both extremely enjoy watching movies, and there is a free movie channel provided to patients.

Kevin and I just got done watching a movie called *All About the Morgans*. It was a great show! For that hour and a half, we relaxed, had fun, laughed, and smiled at each other. It felt like we were someplace other than the clinic. Once the movie was over, I looked around and thought, *Oh, that's right. We're at the Mayo Clinic.*

This took our minds off of everything, and it felt really good, even if it was only for a short while.

After the movie, I needed to leave so Kevin could rest for a while.

I know these e-mails are long, but I really need to write them as I do. It helps me to understand what's going on by typing details. It helps my memory, gives me something to do, is therapy for me, let's others know the details so they don't feel left in the dark, and helps me to feel inside my heart to express myself.

You know, being down at the Mayo had made me realize some things. I have been reminded lately of the beauty of what's around us. Are we *really* aware of the architecture, signs history, etc., of our town or neighborhood? Wouldn't the local museum be interesting? Why don't we take the time to look and pay attention? That is my goal when I get back home in Howard Lake. In fact, our local newspaper has a contest of a mystery picture. A picture is taken the previous week of a part of a sign, marker, business, etc. The first one to call with the correct answer as to what it is wins. I never know the answer.

I also am trying to appreciate what was and is. Not of what's to come. I used to spend *so many hours* working and trying to do something that wasn't in God's plans. Yes, I even knew that it wasn't meant for me to do. I continued to do them just the same and even tried to make a deal with God, to change his mind. I did what I wanted anyway.

Guess what! The plan God had for me is what I'm doing right now, at this moment. I am loving my husband and *trying* to be a mother and caretaker of my family.

No matter what obstacle is in our way, God doesn't let us have things on our shoulders that we can't fix or handle.

All of this enlightenment is good for me, but I feel that the most important of all is accepting God's answers to our prayers, whether it's what we asked for or not.

WEDNESDAY, JULY 14, 2010, 2:20 P.M., DAY 9

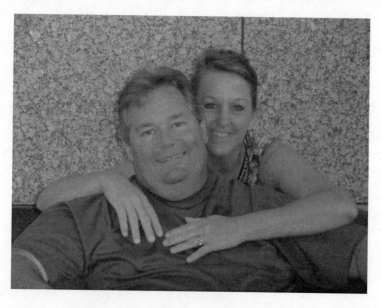

Kevin and I between appointments.

Kevin didn't sleep much last night at all. He still feels pretty good, but the nurses told him to take Imodium and Tylenol PM anyway.

The doctor's told us that Kevin extracted 2,700 cells yesterday. This made the doctors very happy. The nurses told us to plan on Kevin to be extracting cells every day until Sunday.

We are expecting our two daughters to arrive here soon in Rochester to stay overnight and spend some time with us. I am so anxious to see them, and I have so much to tell them and show them. I had asked them a few days earlier to bring beans and other produce from our garden down with them. I have been craving fresh garden vegetables and would like to share them with others at the Gift of Life House.

They are going to stay overnight in the hotel next to the clinic. I wish we could stay with them but Kevin is comfortable at the Gift House and I need to be with him at all times. The girls really needed some time alone together anyway. This separation has been tough on Stephanie. Both of them are excited to hear that they will be on their own at times and have access to a pool and hot tub in the hotel.

After I wrote the e-mail yesterday, I felt that I wanted to clarify something to those of you who don't know me very well. I am very blessed to be able to be stay home to be a housewife. I don't just sit in the house reading books and go out for coffee. Not that that's bad or anything, I am just not personally able to do that. I was also blessed with a gift to talk and serve and love people. I waitress for a *wonderful* seasonal orchard restaurant in Winsted called Carlson's Apple Orchard. I sell Mary Kay cosmetics to my customers, raise chickens in the summer, have a huge garden and I am also involved with the community.

I don't know why but I wanted to clarify this because you know how it goes. Some people/adults feel at times that the grass is always greener on the other side even when we don't know the details of the other side.

Tomorrow is the same schedule for us. The girls will take turns sitting with Kevin while he is in collection. When one girl is with Kevin, the other one will be with me. I plan on showing them the wonderful activities that go on in Rochester on Thursdays. They have what's called "Thursdays on First." It's like a flea market with all sorts of food and crafts. This is located within the Mayo buildings and down First Street. There is also entertainment throughout the day. I really enjoy this and can't wait until Kevin feels good enough to do this with me too.

God bless and will e-mail again soon.

THURSDAY, JULY 15, 2010, DAY 10

We had a very nice night last night with our two girls. It's too bad that they forgot the vegetables from our garden. Some of the guests at our gift house and I were looking forward to fresh produce. Oh, well, the growing season has just begun and they can bring them next time they visit.

After breakfast at the hotel with the girls, Kevin did his normal appointments for the day. Notice, I said Kevin instead of us. The girls and I spent about three hours going through Thursdays on First here in Rochester. I took a lot of pictures, and we took in some history. We saw the first ambulance used at the Mayo Clinic, saw wonderful art displays, and visited the historic playhouse, which is now turned in to a Barnes & Noble book store. We had a wonderful time being together relaxing.

Kaylee told us that this trip to see us helped her deal with this whole situation better. She felt that what helped was being able to see that we are okay. She was personally able to see Kevin and touch and hug him. Both girls were comforted with more facts about the treatment process. It is always easier to understand if you can actually see the process as it is being explained than just hearing it.

Good news! Kevin extracted twelve million stem cells in three days! He doesn't need to go early in the morning tomorrow! He is *so happy* to be done with that step in the process! He says that even with his fat belly, the doctors and nurses are running out of room to poke the needle for his blood-thinner medicine and the original primer shot. He has so many black and blue marks.

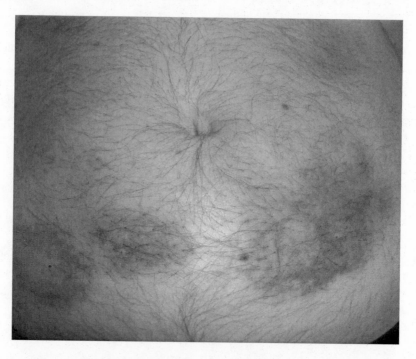

Underneath some of the black and blue spots are hard lumps. The nurse told us the reason for the hardness under the bruises often occurs when the bruises get repunctured and heal from the inside. We still need to keep watch because we had a number of instances that he started bleeding in those spots during evening hours.

The doctors will be calling us in the morning to let us know what our new schedule is. Until then, I have nothing else of importance to tell you, but I do have a funny and/ or stupid story to share.

This afternoon, I wasn't able to get out of the bathroom in the subway. I pulled on the handle, and it wouldn't budge. I knew there was another person in the same bathroom but was still in the stall. I said out loud in a concerned voice, "Oh, no! We're stuck! I think we're locked in!" I kept trying to pull the door. I was hoping to get it open before the other person came out of her stall. I didn't want her to be frightened. I checked and knew it was a pull, not a push. Again, I said, "Seriously, we're locked in. Now what are we going to do?!" The other lady came out of the stall with a little smirk on her face, washed her hands, went to the door handle, and turned it to open. Boy did I ever feel stupid! I told her, "I knew my brain wasn't working today!"

The good news about that is that when I told Kevin and the girls what had happened, they all laughed so hard. Kaylee noticed how much this had lightened Kevin's mood.

We are praying for treatment to continue with no setbacks. That the side effects Kevin gets, if any, are minimal.

FRIDAY, JULY 16, 11:56 P.M.

We would have been able to sleep in today because we didn't have any morning appointments. You know how that goes, when you can sleep in, you get up earlier than if you had to get up.

It was a beautiful day here as far as the weather, and Kevin is feeling pretty good. The diarrhea he has been having is slowing down but Kevin can still feel the little guys, cells, working his joints. He has quite a few aches.

I'm so glad that I heard my cell phone at 7:00 p.m. tonight. Evidentially, the blood draw done earlier today showed Kevin's blood thickness was not what they needed it to be. We were told that we needed to come down to the clinic to get the Fragmen shot right away. Fragmen is a blood thinner. The doctors want Kevin to continue this shot for now until further notice.

This has just changed our weekend schedule. Saturday we have an appointment for the blood-thinner shot. On Sunday, they will do the added shots and blood test at the same time as our already scheduled appointment. We already had an appointment at three thirty to flush Kevin's catheter lines.

Our schedule for Monday is four appointments with the coordinators and the doctors to discuss the transplant process. We are hoping to start the chemotherapy on Tuesday. If nothing gets in the way, we will have chemo on Tuesday and Wednesday. Then we are planning on the cell transplant on Thursday.

We have been told that patients usually get sick around the fifth day after the chemo has started and usually lasts seven to ten days. We have seen patients at the Gift of Life House, as they were already going through this stage of treatment. Some have been really sick, have fainted and some that needed to be hospitalized. We have seen them come back from the hospital and have gone home because they were once again healthy. Some had a quick turn around, and others had a tougher time recovering.

We were told by the doctors that it is good for Kevin to have a couple of days off. Blood-thinner shot appointments and flushing his tubes once is enough for the weekend. We need to have his body regroup before the next step because the next step is very stressful on the body.

I will keep in touch with each one of you and ask for your continued prayers. I probably won't e-mail again until Monday unless something else comes up. I need to take the weekend off too.

MONDAY, JULY 19, DAY 14

Hope you all had a wonderful weekend.

My mom and dad came down to visit with us yesterday. We all had such a wonderful time visiting and watching the Twins game.

Kevin had a blood-thinner shot at the clinic. Then we had a meeting with the transplant coordinator and hematology and transplant doctor to go over some last-minute details.

Kevin passed everything and will start his chemotherapy tomorrow. This is what we were hoping for.

I will e-mail tomorrow to let you all know more about this and how Kevin did.

TUESDAY, JULY 20, 2010, 5:09 P.M., DAY 15—KEVIN −2

Please keep in your prayers my great grandmother Elsie Sauter. She is ninety-six years old and was taken to the hospital in Waconia this morning with a fever and dehydration and was diagnosed with pneumonia. I love her so much! I hope nothing bad happens to her. I'm so far away and feel the need to see her.

The e-mails from here on out will be numbered starting with −2 for today, −1 for tomorrow, and 0 for Thursday. On Thursday, the day will be 0 because this is a new day for Kevin because he is getting his healthier cells put back in his bloodstream. We will count positive numbers from here on out to say how many days Kevin is in remission. Isn't this great?

I changed Kevin's catheter bandage this morning. It seemed easier when I had an instructor watching and helping me. We had a nurse look at the bandage at our first appointment today. I was told that it looked good and that it will get easier to change each time I do it. I wanted a nurse to check it because it is so important to do this well. There is a chance of infection if the bandage isn't sealed correctly.

Today, Kevin had his blood-thinner shot and his first chemotherapy treatment. This only took about three hours for this whole appointment. We picked up the medication that Kevin was prescribed to take during this procedure. These medications will help to relieve some of the side effects from the chemotherapy.

We also needed to pick up tools for brushing his teeth and special soap for the shower. They don't want chemo patients to brush teeth with a toothbrush. The bristles might tear his gums, causing him to bleed so he needs to use a sponge. We definitely don't want him to bleed. He also was prescribed special mouth rinses to help prevent too many mouth sores.

The chemo treatment might irritate his skin, so he was told he needed to wash with basis soap. This soap is for sensitive skin with chamomile. He told me that when he was young, his mother always bought this soap for them to use.

Being as chemo could possibly irritate the skin, I had scheduled a dermatologist appointment tomorrow for Kevin at the clinic. I thought it was necessary for Kevin to have the redness on his face and spots on his legs checked out now. This way, there would be a record of how these issues of redness and rash were already before any side effects would occur. The spots on his legs appeared seven to ten years ago. He was told by our family doctor that these could be from excess fluid.

We are both doing fine right now, trying to learn everything that we can. Disinfecting everything we touch and catching ourselves in old habits. We can't kiss or anything right now because of germs. No smack or nothing! This is really different because we give each other a kiss every morning and most nights.

We met a woman today that is back at the Mayo with her husband. He had received a transplant two and a half years ago and is reinfected with cancer. He needed another transplant. The difference between his and Kevin's procedure is that this man needed donor cells because they couldn't use his own for one reason or another. The human body sometimes doesn't accept foreign objects. Foreign objects like cadaver bones, donor cells, donor marrow, or anything that is received from someone other than you.

This woman also said that two years ago, when they were here at the Mayo Clinic, they stayed in the Gift of Life Transplant House. A virus got in the house, and people got really sick. This was the same house that we are all staying in now. How sad and scary this must have been for everyone.

This woman was even sent home away from her husband, who was there for treatment, because she caught the virus. Hers had turned into pneumonia. After the doctor cleared her from this, she was able to come back to be with her husband.

Each year, more and more is learned in the medical field and what we need to do in order to prevent illnesses. Daily living includes dealing with germs, cleaning, disinfecting, food choices, side effects, and more. We need to stay aware of our surroundings and the things we use. We should be thinking of others who could get infected from us and our germs. I have been watching others and noticing things that I don't like. I have decided that I need to clean an area before I even touch it. This way, if they didn't disinfect when they were done, I will do it before I touch it and infects me.

WEDNESDAY, JULY 21, DAY 16—KEVIN −1

After the dermatology appointment today, we will go for Kevin's second chemo treatment and shot.

There is a newer sewing machine here at the Gift of Life House for guests to use. I needed something constructive to do to occupy my mind and time. I decided to see if I remember how to sew. I found a free pattern online for do-rags for cancer patients I got some brown material, and after some frustration and time, I had completed one. It didn't look very nice, but it would serve the purpose in keeping the head warm.

Yesterday afternoon, I'll be honest that I was flustered, afraid, felt like I needed some air, needed to scream, and needed to cry, but I couldn't. I was thinking about the weeks to come. We've been listening to others, and learning that *nobody* is the same as far as treatment goes. Even if it's the same disease; everyone has a different process of medical help. The only thing that is in common is feeling extremely sick, puking, nausea, not wanting to eat, not hungry, dehydration, sores in the mouth and throat, trouble swallowing, tired, etc. Sixty percent of patients end up in the hospital to get help with fluids and whatever is necessary to keep their body functioning.

Now, I do know that that doesn't mean Kevin will get like that and I won't be afraid anymore. At the same time, I need to think about how important it is to not forget anything that we've learned. I also am trying to get myself psyched up to keep Kevin's spirits up.

Even today, something I thought I needed to do was wrong. I thought it was necessary for sanitation to wash fruit/vegetables with soap and water. NO! The doctor's said not to do that! You will make more bacteria. You are to only wash foods you eat with water. Use the force from the water or use a soft brush and scrub the food while the water is running. When we purchase lettuce that says on the bag that it's prewashed already, don't rewash it! You will make bacteria on the lettuce. Open the bag and eat it.

There is a woman here from Arkansas who is as sweet as can be. She has a disease that is very rare. They are trying to treat it with a possible kidney transplant. Her skin is discolored yellow with jaundice. Her finger and toe muscles will often tighten up. When this happens, her fingers curl in toward her palm and her toes curl toward her heels. It looks very painful and like she has rheumatoid arthritis with her curled fingers. It is very difficult for her to walk at times and hang on to anything because she also doesn't have much strength. She also has difficulty opening things because she can't open her fingers. I was so fortunate to be able to help her today.

At therapy, she was told that she needs to start using a paraffin wax heater. It heats up wax, you put your hands or feet in there for a couple of minutes, and then you take them out. Your hands are nice and warm, and it feels so good. Then you peel the wax off after awhile. The doctors want her to do that before her therapy appointment because this will make it easier for them to stretch her muscles and manipulate them due to her muscles being warm. She told me that it would be really good for people with arthritis to do this too. For those of us with arthritis, maybe we should try this. I just know that she told me that the cheap machines don't heat up as good and you get what you pay for.

How humbled I am. This woman is filled with love and faith. She keeps going no matter what is in front of her. She is waiting for a kidney donor to match and is not having any success. She is again on a waiting list. That must make her feel so helpless.

It's plain to see that God has blessed the Mayo Clinic. They display pictures of Jesus in almost every room we've been in while in the hospital for treatments. My favorite picture is a patient on the table with a nurse and doctor tending to her with Jesus by their side.

Kevin needs to wear a face mask constantly now to help protect him from any airborne germs. The only place he doesn't need it on is in our room at the Gift of Life House and a disinfected patient room at the clinic. Our bedroom had been disinfected before we arrived, and I was to keep it disinfected during our stay. This mask makes Kevin *really* hot and uncomfortable.

We are going to find a barber for Kevin's hair to be cut really short today. It seems as if Kevin is not okay with losing his hair. We both felt that it would be much easier on him to lose it when it's shorter. It won't be as drastic of a change then or as noticeable. I am hoping that this will also keep him cooler. The beautician told us that when customers come in for the head shave due to illness, women have a much better attitude about this than men. I will continue to pray for calmness, healing, thanksgiving, comfort, courage, kindness, and patience for you, myself, and Kevin during this time. Everyone deals with struggles from time to time. They are different in severity and topic but nonetheless are trials for us all.

Each day we can make a difference, if not for someone else, how about for ourselves? God bless!

WEDNESDAY, JULY 21, DAY 16 — KEVIN −1, SECOND E-MAIL

I thought I'd fill you in on the chemotherapy treatment Kevin is receiving. I have been asked some questions in the past in regard to this, and I hope this clears some of them up.

Chemotherapy is designed to kill fast-growing cancer cells. It can *also* affect healthy cells that grow quickly. These include cells that line your mouth, intestines; cells in your bone marrow that make blood cells, and cells that make your hair grow. Chemotherapy causes side effects when it harms these healthy cells. The amount of side effects you get and how long they last depends on the type of cancer you have and the type of chemo you receive.

Sometimes, chemo causes long-term side effects that don't go away. These may include damage to your heart, lungs, nerves, kidneys, or reproductive organs. Some chemo may cause a second cancer years later. We are *not* going to worry or concern ourselves with this.

Doctors have many ways to prevent or treat chemotherapy side effects and help patients heal after each treatment session.

Kevin already has medicines (I believe nine or ten prescriptions) to help alleviate these side effects. I do have a chart telling me about specific side effects and ways we can manage them. Examples are mouth sores: Kevin needs to chew on ice *a lot*. This will also keep his mouth cooler. Anemia: rest, etc. Appetite changes: eat five or six small meals or snacks each day instead of three bigger meals, etc. Bleeding: blow your nose gently, etc. Infection: wash hands often, etc. Mouth and throat changes: check your mouth and tongue every day, etc. Nausea and vomiting: have foods and drinks that are warm or cool (not hot or cold), etc. Plus there are more, but I think you've heard enough.

As soon as I get together a list of things I need to remember for sanitary purposes and cleanliness, I will forward them to you. It's nice to have a list if you, like me, need to or want to start doing them at home also.

Remember, it will be Kevin's day 0 tomorrow! He is getting his transplant in the hospital. This will take approximately ten hours or so for this procedure.

As you all know, no matter what is going on in your life, reality continues. Are the kids in denial or troubled with what's going on? I don't know at this point yet, but they have not even been calling me to check on how things are going. Each time I have been calling home, the kids don't have any time for me. They feel like I'm checking up on them. They have been too busy for me. It's like I'm interrupting their freedom, time with their friends, and outings.

THURSDAY, JULY 22, 11:59 A.M., KEVIN DAY 0

Good news! My great grandma is home from the hospital, and I want to thank you all for your thoughts and prayers. She is doing well and feeling a lot better. This is a huge relief to our whole family.

This morning, we needed to be at the hospital at 5:30 a.m. for the transplant process. Before the doctors could give Kevin his stem cells, they needed to give him fluids. These fluids will help his body prepare for the transplant and help to deal with the type of preservative that is in the cells bag. This type of fluid is used to protect the cells during the frozen stage. The fluids are administered through an IV to the intake port of the catheter. This process took four hours to complete. After that, Kevin was given four million stem cells back. These were some of the cells from his cell collection last week.

At first, the transplant was going too fast. Kevin became flushed and really hot. The nurses needed to slow the process down and put cold compresses on his forehead for a short while to get his temperature back down. After one hour of the transplant, the doctors needed to give Kevin more fluid for four more hours for the same reason as earlier.

We will continue to come in as an outpatient for daily checkups. Kevin's transplant came out very well. We are praying for God's healing power to make sure the cells reattach and multiply. If they don't attach, this means that his body is not accepting his own cells back into his system. If this is the case, he will need a donor for a new transplant. The doctors should know this in about seven to ten days. Thank you for sending your replies, prayers, and support during this journey.

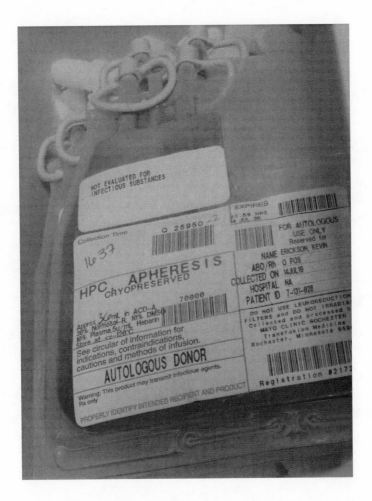

This is a frozen bag of cells. Kevin received four of these today. The label on top is read very carefully to make sure it's Kevin's cell pack.

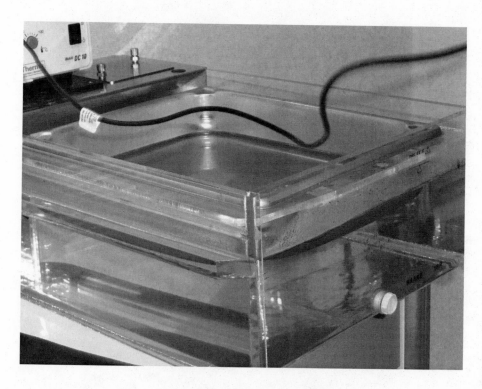

This is the warmer that is set to thirty-eight degrees.

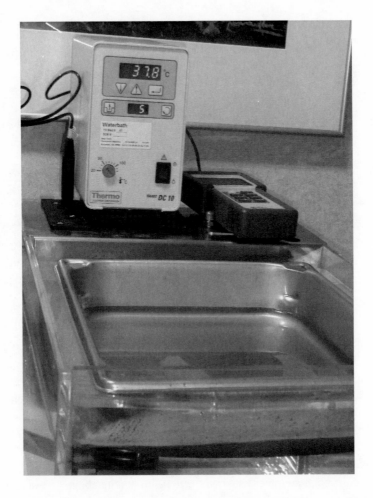

Notice the thermometer on the front, top. This warmer thaws the cells from the frozen stage and prepares them for the transplant.

This is a copy of all of the records they create from the cell harvest.

FRIDAY, JULY 23, DAY 1

This morning, Kevin told me, "If I feel this bad right now, I'm in trouble next week." He has some nausea, is really tired, and has no energy.

Parking on the streets and by parking meters is free all night in Rochester until 8:00 a.m. Yesterday I put quarters in the parking meter at 8:00 a.m. I planned on leaving the hospital at 9:30 a.m., so I put in $1.50 for one and a half hours. When I came out at 9:30 a.m. to go, I found a ticket on my windshield. The ticket was for $17.00. It showed that it was written out at 8:48 a.m. This didn't make sense to me at all that I should have had a ticket.

I called the phone number listed on the ticket to inquire about it. I was informed that the meter I used was only good for half an hour no matter how much money I put into it. I told her that I had never used a meter before and wondered where my $1.50 went. She laughed and said, "You're in the big city now, so you'll have to pay attention next time and look on the very top of the meter. It will tell you if it's a half-hour meter or ninety-minute meter." She did let me off the ticket, and I didn't have to pay. I felt stupid that I didn't know about meters. I learned something new again!

Each day, as of now, we will need to be seen in the outpatient department at the hospital at 9:30 a.m. At this appointment, the medical staff will check to make sure

Kevin is getting enough fluids, check his heart and his overall health issues, and do blood checks. I need to keep track daily of Kevin's temperature, the medications taken, the amounts and the time they are taken for the doctors to review. I also need to keep a journal of the foods he is eating and the fluids he drinks. The medical staff checks my notes daily at our appointments. We also have a dietician come in to check on the lists every once in a while.

I will not e-mail until next week unless something else comes up. Have a great weekend.

FRIDAY, JULY 23, DAY 1, SECOND E-MAIL

Kevin's taste buds have already started to change. Even water doesn't taste good to Kevin anymore. It's a good thing there's a variety of liquids to drink which makes it easier for him to get the necessary daily fluids.

Kevin's sleeping right now yet and it's late at night. I wanted to talk to someone about what I've been thinking about, so why not the computer?

Today, I visited with an elderly woman from Virginia who is here with her boyfriend of twenty years. When her boyfriend told her that he was coming to the Mayo Clinic for a heart and lung transplant, he told her that he was only scheduled here for two weeks. When she asked about his caregivers, he said that he was coming alone because his children wouldn't come. Well, she thought she could handle living with him and caring for him for two weeks and came with him. Evidently they don't live together because they don't cohabitate well but still love each other.

Well, she has been here since May or something and has been struggling for some time now. I asked her if his children ever did come to give her a break from the caregiver role, and she told me, "You know, family problems? Well, there you go. Everyone has them." I am assuming that this is the case here. I have been thinking about this topic from time to time ever since Kevin got ill.

In a previous e-mail, I told you that when we found out that Kevin had cancer, it suddenly became easier to let the little things that would normally get to me bounce off of me more. I also shared of how this has changed our lives. Kevin and I definitely appreciate each other more, want to spend quality time together more, etc. I think it was Kevin's dad who has always said this, but Kevin also says it. "If I don't see or spend time with someone while they are alive, why should I go to the funeral when they die, unless I want to support the family?" Isn't that true?

How many times do you see or hear on the news about the people who have died in a crash, got shot from the police, etc? When the family and/or friends are interviewed, they all say how nice they were. How everyone liked this person. How they wouldn't have ever done anything wrong to get shot. How it must be someone else's fault. Not mentioning that they got shot because they were caught and ran away or anything you know. Also it is said what bright students they were, etc. How many times, I wonder, were these individuals that passed away actually told these things and felt appreciated or liked while they were alive by these people who were interviewed?

Maybe I'm wrong, but my point is this. Now is the time to open our mouths to those we love. Truly forgive those who have wronged us or people we love and try to spend time with others before it is too late. Sometimes I know it's a hard thing to do. Some people just have a hard time complimenting others, and everyone's got such busy lives. Sometimes our pride gets in our way, and we say, "Why should I forgive? I didn't do anything wrong. It's their fault, not mine." We still need to find a way to fix it or at least take care of our end in the forgiving process.

In my past, there were a few people that I had a *very* difficult time forgiving. Some for mental and physical abuse, for saying things about my family, for judging me, for not letting me participate, for not letting me be their friend, for controlling me, for being snotty, etc. One night, a few years ago, we watched a movie or saw something on TV about someone who was raped or kept captive. I don't really remember which it was. I do know that it was very disturbing to me. You see, I could relate to this situation. The next morning, I couldn't stop crying. I tried everything and nothing worked. I didn't know what to do. I called the church and told them what was happening, and they told me to come in right away for prayer ministry.

I had police records from the night I was raped fourteen years ago. I had saved these records in a file and never looked at them again. I kept transporting them with me everywhere I had relocated throughout the years. I guess I felt that if I ever needed to prove my innocence to anyone at any time, I would be able to show them the police report. I was surprised that the first thing I needed to do before I went to church was get this report. I wanted to prove my innocence to Pastor Joel and whoever else was there. I knew *exactly* where it was. With the memory issues I have, this has baffled me ever since that I always knew where these reports were.

When I arrived in the church office, I handed the rape report to Pastor Joel. He told me he didn't want to read the report. I was very disappointed at first that he didn't want to read or even look at them. I mean, I saved this for fourteen years! This is the day I can prove my innocence.

I realized during this ministry session that it was not just the rapist that I needed to forgive. I needed to forgive family and friends who questioned my innocence. I also needed to forgive myself for being angry at them and also for being angry at myself. There were many times that I thought, "What if I'd have done this or that?" I mean the police told me that I did the right thing. This man had a record already. I needed to forgive everyone, not just some. I needed to put it *all* at the foot of the cross. I was able to stop crying during this time, and it was like the details on the records had disappeared. It didn't matter what the report said anymore, and it hasn't bothered me again since then.

At the end of our time, Pastor Joel asked if I could throw the reports away, and I did. Wow! Fourteen years and in the course of one and a half hours, I was fine to remove it from my life. There was no reason to keep it. I didn't have to prove my innocence to anyone. God knows the truth and that's all that matters. I wasn't getting the forgiving thing done on my own. Deep down, this had caused me stress, grief, and resentment at times for years. With prayer ministry, I learned how to forgive by just putting my issues at the foot of the cross and I let God take them from me. I still need to be reminded of this process from time to time and actually still find it difficult to do many times. Prayer ministry will be different for everyone, but it has really helped me in so many ways in my life.

Just in case you do or don't know. If you say, "I forgive you" or "I forgive my neighbor," but do not truly forgive, God and others can tell. So don't try to fool yourself. What I'm trying to get at is that if you and a family member or friend are having relationship issues, it's not too late. Get it fixed right now before it's too late. Before they get sick or things get worse. Please don't have any regrets in your life. Not everyone needs to like everyone, but family is family. If you forgive, please truly forgive, or it is pointless and worthless. Jesus didn't just *say* he forgave us. He *truly* forgave us and doesn't hold anything against us if we do wrong to him. He only forgives us again because of his love for us.

I pray that Kevin's health is restored and we live many years together. I also pray that this e-mail might make a difference to someone's life who is reading this. I know it made me open my eyes again right now. Thank you for reading my long e-mails.

SATURDAY, JULY 31, 11:24 A.M., KEVIN DAY 9

Please pray for my grandma Elsie again. She's back in the hospital because she is dehydrated and still has a little bit of pneumonia. I know it's been a while since my last e-mail. It's been a weird week for me. I am trying to keep Kevin as comfortable as I can. Our friends Mike and Pete came to visit this last Sunday, and it was really nice to see them again.

I was told that some people have commented that they don't like reading about God all of the time. My e-mails are getting too religious for them. How in the world can I tell of the miracles to everyone without mentioning the truth!

This bothered Kevin and I a little bit. I won't let that deter me from writing like I have been. I can't. I need and want to express my faith and desires. If someone doesn't like it, then don't read it.

Monday, I took Kevin for a haircut and shave at the salon at Walmart. We have been told that it's just a matter of time before he loses all of his hair, and we know he is concerned about being bald. While he was waiting for his stylist, I went shopping in the store for a few things that we needed at the house. Well, when I returned to the salon, the stylist was almost finished. Kevin got only two inches cut off his head. I commented and showed my disapproval. He told me that this was short enough. I didn't realize how hard this would be for him to do.

Tuesday, Kevin had a really rough day not feeling well at all. At this time, Kevin hasn't thrown up yet or has had any mouth or throat sores to speak of either yet. He just had no energy to do anything, which is normal at this stage of treatment. Kevin still has minimal cell count left. The cells that he got transplanted have not joined in the marrow yet. Kevin knows that he *needs* to eat and drink in order to get better and stay out of the hospital. He has been forcing as much food at mealtime and drinking as many liquids as he can drink as possible. It's getting harder and harder each day to keep this up due to his loss of appetite and nausea. When someone feels like this, nothing even looks appetizing either.

Even being so, the doctor's told Kevin on Thursday that he is a spectacular transplant patient. He is doing better than most this far along in the stage of treatment. Kevin felt so good about that report that now he doesn't think he will lose his hair at all. He had told this to a couple of people at the transplant house already. My bet is on day 17 or so, his hair will be falling out.

Last night, when I took Kevin's temperature, it was normal. This morning I took his temperature and it was 99.4 degrees. When we got to the hospital for his blood draw at 9:30 a.m., it was 100.3. It is creeping up, so the doctors decided to take blood cultures to see if there is an infection. If there is, they would need to pinpoint it as soon as possible so they can treat it appropriately.

One blood draw was taken from his arm and one from his catheter. They are currently giving him two types of antibiotics just in case it's an infection. They are also waiting to see how his platelet count is to see if he needs another dose of platelets. Kevin already received platelets yesterday afternoon because his count was low.

Kevin and I both are so grateful to be here together. This morning as we were walking, I was thinking how much I really love this man. There is no other like him, that's for sure. He's perfect for me because he is honest as can be. He says it like it is and no other way. He is patient, giving, reasonable, and true, and he is a great father for our children. I noticed again this past week of his determination and positive attitude to beat this cancer. He has no doubt that he will be healed.

Take care and have a great weekend.

JULY 31, 2010, 8:21 P.M., DAY 9, SECOND E-MAIL

This past Sunday was the Ronald McDonald fundraiser in Rochester. I had always heard of the Ronald Mcdonald House but never really paid too much attention as to find out facts. This house is just a few doors down from the transplant house that Kevin and I are currently staying at. The Ronald McDonald House has forty-eight rooms for patients, and each patient can have up to five family members stay with them. There is a minimum charge per night to help reduce costs to the families just like where we are staying. This makes it affordable for everyone. Some patients can and will pay more to stay there and some can only pay the minimal.

The fundraiser they had for this house was a motorcycle bike ride. I'm not sure where the cycles met up before they traveled to Rochester. Maybe they even met somewhere in Rochester, but when they arrived, you sure heard them.

There were 1,450 motorcycles, and $119,045.00 was raised. This is phenomenal! Kevin told me that I could go down to check out the event. He said he'd be okay to be alone for a little while. I was surprised to see that there was a group of bagpipe players, an ice cream social, greeters around the area, and another band coming later in the day. There were quite a few people participating and supporting this effort.

I also noticed something that made my eyes jump out of the socket. Now you might think I'm kidding about this but I'm not. I saw a young man that is about ten feet tall. I felt so sorry for him! When I went back to the house, I had told some people what I saw. I was hoping to express to them that there is always someone worse off than all of us.

Can you imagine how he gets stared at? How children might be scared when they see him? How some people would walk away or around him for fear? How he gets teased from smart alecks? We all can take medicine for our illnesses, and most people can't even tell if someone is sick or anything. Well, this young man can't hide from his illness or get medicines to make it go away.

I talked to the janitor at the Gift House, and he told me that this young man grew up in Russia. He had come to the Ronald McDonald House in Rochester years earlier because of his disease. This disease was very rare, and it didn't allow him to stop growing. I was also told that he is a really nice young man and he and his family decided to move to Rochester.

We all need to take a good look when we are sad and disappointed about our looks, body shapes, hair color, etc., and see what blessings we do have. This young man was blessed with kindness and gentleness to show people that it's not what's on the outside but on the inside that counts.

Kevin is in the hospital two times each day for a while now. This is due to requiring antibiotics and extra platelets. When his cell count is low, he needs infusion of platelets.

I have been getting a few phone calls from Stephanie every once in a while. She is really sad. She misses home and doesn't like her situation. I felt so bad for her. I told her that she could come home for only a couple of days. We felt it was the best thing for her to stay where she was at because she would get picked on at home. I tried to reassure her that it won't be long yet and things will get better for her.

Sanitation List

Here is a list of sanitary things that I've learned from this Mayo trip. You probably know all of these, but I need a list anyway to hang up at home.

Don't wash fruit with soap. Just wash with water with friction or a scrub brush. I was told that there is a recipe for fruit wash from the University of Minnesota on Google.com.

Have the well water checked at home.

Wipe off with disinfectant wipes all tops of cans before opening.

Refrigerate butter. It is not suggested to store on butter on the counter or on the table.

When washing your hands, hand sanitizer is just as good as, if not better than, antibacterial soap. When hands are cracked from too much washing, bacteria can stay in the cracks of the skin.

Don't wipe counter with dishcloths. This will infect whatever you wipe with bacteria from the dishes. Use a paper towel or disinfectant towel or wipe instead.

Have fresh Dixie cups to rinse mouth after brushing teeth instead of a cup.

Ask for a straw with the paper on when ordering all beverages. You don't know what handled the rim of the cup, where it sat, or what it sat on before it got to your table. And watch your waitress as to where she carries the cup. You don't know if she was just handling dirty dishes or not.

Don't drink from stir straws with no paper on it. Do you know how many hands touched them trying to get one out?

Flush toilet with the opposite hand that you use to wipe your bottom with.

I don't want to become a germ phobic, but I do realize that there are some things that I need to change at my home to keep things as sanitary as possible for Kevin.

Kevin's immune system needs to start completely over. He even needs to get all of his baby shots taken over in one year.

I would like to pass on this prayer that was given to Kevin from a friend.

I said a prayer for you today, and know God must have heard I felt the answer in my heart, although he spoke no word! I didn't ask for wealth or fame, I knew you wouldn't mind.

I asked him to send treasures of a far more lasting kind! I asked that he'd be near you at the start of each new day. To grant you health and blessings and friends to share your way! I asked for happiness for you in all things great and small. But, it was for his loving care I prayed the most of all!

Take care and I will probably send an update in a few days. As of right now, Kevin doesn't feel very well at all. Most of the cancer patients that we've met have gone through something like this. You need to hit bottom in order to climb to the top. We're not sure if this is the bottom yet, but Kevin has the right attitude for this journey.

SUNDAY, AUGUST 1, 2010, 2:21 P.M.,
FIRST E-MAIL, DAY 10

We went in to the hospital at 7:00 a.m. for Kevin's blood draw and antibiotic IV. We were updated on the tests that are completed at this time.

Kevin does *not* have an infection. His recent temperature *could* have been high for a number of reasons. Now that the necessary tests were done and the results were good, doctors are not concerned at all. It's been common for fevers to develop in this type of procedure.

Kevin's platelet count, clotting cells, were good today. Because of this, he doesn't need an IV for that. It's very possible that he will need this a different day though. We'll take one day at a time.

We were informed that Kevin's left ventricle of his heart is larger than his right ventricle. This is probably due to having high blood pressure. We were also told that due to Kevin's drop in hemoglobin, this would put strain on the heart, which could make the heart beat irregular. Because of this, tonight while Kevin gets another dose of antibiotics, he will also get a blood transfusion.

Kevin doesn't feel very good again today. Early this afternoon, I thought he looked flushed and hot. I took his temperature. It was 103.4. I panicked and called the hospital. They said that there is nothing they can do for Kevin at the moment. This is because he is already on an antibiotic schedule, and they can't change the time of treatment. They can only give antibiotic ten hours apart, and there's nothing else they can do. They told me to just give him Tylenol. One hour later, his temperature went down to 102.3. I was relieved and thought this was due to the Tylenol.

His appointment tonight is at 7:00 p.m., and it will take about two hours or so for this. He is *not* eating very well at all. He is cold, sweaty, and burning up. He continues to have a positive attitude even through all of this. I can plainly see the pain and the agony that he is enduring. He isn't a man who likes to complain. He says, "Hey, this is the process. There are many people who are a lot sicker than me." What a stud!

Take care.

SUNDAY, AUGUST 1, 2010
(update typed MONDAY, AUGUST 2, 2:31 A.M.)

Day 10, ICU 1, second e-mail

It was so difficult for me to see Kevin in so much pain. There is a recliner upstairs in the Gift of Life House that is very comfortable for Kevin. It gives the support he needs for his neck. We watched TV and tried to keep our minds occupied until our evening appointment. The room we were in had a lot of windows, and the sunshine felt really good.

Mid afternoon, I took his temperature again and it was higher, so I called the hospital again to ask if I could bring him in. I felt that he needed extra care that I wasn't providing for him. They told me again that they still wouldn't be able to do anything more for him than I can at the house. The hospital staff told me to continue giving him Tylenol and try to keep him comfortable. They suggested for me to give him a lukewarm shower to cool his body temp down at this point. The only way they would want to see him before his regularly scheduled appointment is if he would start to shiver.

It was a really long day to say the least. We never thought 7:00pm would come soon enough.

We went in for our normally scheduled appointment in the evening. The nurse came in and started taking Kevin's temperature. She told me that she had doubts that I took Kevin's temperature correctly during the day. She told me that most likely the thermometer I was using was bad. I told her that I took Kevin's temperature many times, and it was always consistent. I wondered why she didn't tell me to use a different thermometer when I had called earlier in the day then. If she had doubts that my information was correct, why didn't she tell me this?

At this time, she took the thermometer from Kevin's mouth and looked stunned when she saw the reading. She didn't say a word to me other than "I'm going to try a different thermometer and see if it's different." When she saw that it was the same, she was very concerned and called the doctor instantly.

Evidentially caregivers call at times with concern about the high temperatures of their loved ones. Most of the times, there is no need of concern and that is why this was handled this way. It was the wrong assumption in this case. Kevin's doctor told him that he is one in a million to react this way. The doctors felt it necessary to take more blood samples to try to pinpoint as to why this was happening.

Kevin and I are both staying at the hospital for the night. The doctors feel that Kevin needs special attention at this point and have moved him to the ICU. The move was due to the challenge of medical staff trying to keep his temperature, breathing, pulse rate, high blood pressure, etc., under control. The doctors weren't able to get his fever below 103 degrees.

Kevin was breathing very hard and had an oxygen mask to help him. The on-call staff was called to come in to do a CT scan on Kevin to try to see what's going on. This scan was ready for him at 11:30 p.m., and I was told that it wouldn't take long. The doctors told me that it takes longer for the travel to and from the scan than it takes to actually do the procedure. Well! One and a half hours later and they still weren't back. Just as I was starting to be overly concerned, they had pulled into the room. I'm sure that they had difficulty with his vitals again.

The next time I saw Kevin, he told me "I remember all of the doctors standing around my bed. I was telling them that I didn't want a catheter. The young doctor with a suit coat said "Mr. Erickson, I don't think you are in any situation to be arguing whether you get a catheter or not. You're getting one."

Please keep us in your prayers. I'll e-mail tomorrow.

MONDAY, AUGUST 2, 2010, 6:46 P.M.

Kevin day 11, ICU 2

Kevin's cells are gone from his bone marrow at this time, and his system has not accepted the cells that were transplanted back to him yet. Because his cells are depleted, this causes him to have no tolerance to bacteria. This is a concern for the doctors and me. He is just miserable! Kevin's hemoglobin, which is a protein that carries oxygen in the red blood cells, is too low. He currently has and is being given blood transfusions at this time to help with that. Kevin's platelets are also low, so he is getting infusion of extra platelets. Platelets will get reduced in number whenever there is a fever like this.

Kevin is also dehydrated at the moment and is getting an infusion of fluids. He has been struggling with drinking enough fluids lately, and the amount of diarrhea he has been dealing doesn't help either. Kevin's breathing pattern is concerning the doctors. He is working way too hard and breathing way too fast. The doctors feel that it is possible that he has fluid in his lungs at this time, which could cause breathing difficulties. They will first give him Lasix in hopes to push out any fluids that could be in the lungs back into the bloodstream. They will try this first just in case this is the reason.

Kevin's temperature has just dropped one degree now, but the doctor thinks that's because the nurses put a cooling blanket under him. The temperature of this blanket is always set at one degree lower than his current body temperature. They change it down as needed due to Kevin's temperature drops.

The doctors are keeping a close watch on him and have him in isolation. There is a possible infection, and they don't have it pinpointed as to what it is yet. To be on the safe side, they are treating it like it could spread or contaminate others. They are giving Kevin an IV of antibiotics that should cover *any* infection type. This can be given ten hours apart. As soon as they can pinpoint what kind of infection it is, then they will target it and try to get rid of it.

Kevin is *very* tired and weak. His hair started to fall out a little bit today. We will get through this first and then worry about shaving his head later.

I don't know if I mentioned this in any previous e-mails. I got in for an appointment at the Mayo Clinic for my head issues. My sister, Penny, volunteered to come to Rochester for my appointment Wednesday morning. My dad will come with her and sit with Kevin while I am gone. He will only do this if Kevin isn't contagious.

The kids are planning on coming down on Thursday, only if Kevin isn't contagious. It is so very hard to see Kevin suffer like this. I don't even know how to explain it to anyone. He is burning up. His face is red. He is sweaty and wet, yet he is cold at times and wants me to cover him up. He is weak, doesn't talk much, and is very uncomfortable. I know a lot of cancer patients go through this and it is part of the process for most, but the doctor told me today that this is a little more intense than usual.

Not to get alarmed. Kevin is in the best place that he can be, and God is with him also.

Take care and I will e-mail again!

TUESDAY, AUGUST 3, 2010, 4:09 A.M.

Day 12, ICU 3

I was told that Kevin's problems may be caused from the high temperature he has now been having for three days. They said this because the CT scan also showed negative to infection. They just need to find out why his temperature is so high. The medical staff wants Kevin to concentrate on his breathing and feel that he needs to be left alone for a while. I went to the family lounge to watch TV in hopes to fall asleep. I finally fell asleep and got a little relief. I woke up at 3:00 a.m. and immediately went to check on Kevin.

He was sleeping but not very sound. His temperature and everything were up again. The nurse asked Kevin if he wanted me to stay. He said that he wanted to try to sleep. The nurse told me to go back to the family lounge and they would come get me if they needed me. I was going to go back to the transplant house to try to get better sleep at that time, but I knew that Kevin wanted me to stay in the hospital. He doesn't want me walking alone at night. I will stay here until 6:30 a.m. and then go to the house for a few hours only if Kevin is in stable condition.

Kevin still had the oxygen mask on, not the breathing tube yet. He looked very uncomfortable. It's plain to see his determination in controlling his breath. It's like he was counting as he was breathing in and pausing between breaths. He was trying to breathe deeply and slowly just like the doctors told him.

Kevin is also *not* under any sedation at this time but has been given morphine. I think they are getting ready to give him another shot of morphine because it did seem to calm him down before.

The doctors are aware that Kevin is a little claustrophobic, but so far, he seems to be fine with that.

I sit here and wonder what Kevin might be thinking right now and how he is feeling. Earlier, I asked him if he was scared, and his answer was "no". He looks so miserable and must be just exhausted because he is working so hard to breathe. I believe this is what Kevin is telling himself throughout this time: "Yea, though I walk through the valleys and the shadows of death, I fear no evil, for thou art with me."

My mom told me the other day what an amazing man Kevin is. I instantly said, "You know, Mom, I married a man just like my dad." He is also very strong, he doesn't complain, is determined, always does the best he can, and will do anything for you if he thinks you need it. My dad is also very firm with his feelings. He isn't very sensitive, and neither is Kevin. Isn't that funny how our lives, attitude, and examples continue on in generations of our family lines to come even in the short time we are here on earth?

I'm getting really tired and will e-mail as soon as I hear any new news. I just want to keep you all updated and ask that you don't worry about us but that you stay strong in your faith and prayers.

TUESDAY, AUGUST 3, 2010, 4:23 A.M.

Day 12, ICU 3, second e-mail

I just went back to Kevin's room to get a couple of pillows for myself. The medical staff was working quickly on Kevin again. It seems like each one of them were so focused on the particular job they had to do in order to save Kevin's life. They were rushing to get him the help he needed.

I just stood outside his room in shock while I watched in horror. I never thought we'd be in this situation. You see and hear about other people going through this but never think it will happen to you. The doctors had to put a breathing tube in Kevin. They felt that he needed more help to breathe than what the mask could do for him. He was working too hard and wasn't stable. They also sedated him a little in hopes to make him more comfortable. His blood pressure isn't handling one of the medicines he is taking very well at all. I heard the nurse quickly order a different one for Kevin.

All I could do was watch and pray. I was so afraid for his life.

TUESDAY, AUGUST 3, 2010, 8:49 A.M.

Day 12, ICU 3, third e-mail

Kevin's temperature started the day out at 105.1. The doctor's were *really* concerned, and they felt that the outlook was grim. I had the feeling that Kevin was going to die today and the children needed to get here as soon as possible to be with us.

Kevin is in *very* critical condition. He has an infection, and they don't know what kind and where it is at this time. Kevin needs help. His internal organs are shutting down. It takes hours for test results to come back from the cultures they took. In the meantime, they have increased his medications in hopes to help matters. They are watching him very carefully right now and doing everything that they can to save his life.

The doctors don't want me with Kevin right now. They need all of the space in the room for medical staff. If another emergency arises, I will be in the way. I can check on him as often as I want from outside the room. In the meantime, I am waiting in the waiting room until the doctors are ready to talk to me. They told me that they will call me when they do their patient rounds to update me on Kevin's condition.

The doctors inquired about the status of our living will and advance directives forms at this time. Kevin had procrastinated on filling these out for weeks. We did, however, manage to get them filled out, but we didn't get them notarized yet. It was necessary for this step to be completed and they instructed me as to where to go for this. Fortunately, I had the proper verification with me and was able to finish the task legally without Kevin. He wasn't coherent at this time and his health is failing. I can't even begin to explain what this made me feel like. It was like giving my husband the death sentence.

I feel helpless. The only new information I have currently received was that they were going to exchange catheters in Kevin. The doctors need an extra port for more medications. The new catheter has three ports, and the one that is already inserted in Kevin only has two ports. There again is a risk for infection during this surgery of insertion. They also don't know if the veins will be open enough to complete this process at this time. They reassured me that there would be multiple attempts, and they would try their hardest in hopes that this will be a successful surgery.

I needed support and family near us at this time. I called Pastor Joel and Mary Lou and asked them to come here. I told them that Kevin is dying, and I needed them. Mary Lou immediately responded with "Karen we're on our way. I'll call you when we get close to Rochester, and we can make a plan to meet so we know where to go."

I notified Kevin's siblings and my family and asked them to pass the information on like usual to everyone. My dad, mom, and brother, Scott, will be bringing our kids, Tony, Kaylee, and Stephanie down here sometime this morning. My sister, Penny, and sister-in-law, Brenda, are coming down later today. With all of these family members, we will be able make arrangements for the kids to either stay down here for a few days or go home. This is extremely important that we are together at this time in our lives.

The night nurse told me this morning, "I'm so impressed with how strong a man Kevin is. I can tell by reading his vitals. His blood pressure and temperature are very high, and his pulse is very rapid. He is so uncomfortable and in so much pain, and he never complains. He just seems so very faithful and calm about the whole thing."

We truly are blessed to have Kevin in our lives and we will stay strong. Staying strong in faith will carry us all through this trial and disease. That's what Kevin would want us to do.

I have been scheduled to see a specialist down here tomorrow for my severe headaches. I truly thought of cancelling this appointment due to Kevin's condition, but decided not to. Kevin definitely would *not* want me to do that. My sister, Penny, will be coming with me to the doctor because I need an extra set of ears and another person to think of questions to ask and take notes. I am not comfortable with my attention span and focus that I would have during this appointment.

We will take each day at a time and know that Kevin is in the very best hands possible.

Again, isn't it something how easy it is to forget making the best of *each* minute we have on earth? To try our hardest and make the best of each situation that we come up against? To spend quality time with loved ones? I have to go now because the doctor called and needs me right now.

TUESDAY, AUGUST 3, 2010, 10:18 A.M.

Day 12, ICU 3, fourth e-mail

The doctors involved in daily patient rounds are ICU doctors and specialists. These rounds are done a couple of times a day to get feedback from other doctor's on each individual case. When there are more ears and minds working and going over a certain case, there are more people that might realize a different method or plan to take care of a situation. There would also be more people to catch something if it might have been missed. I was asked to be with them this morning when they discussed Kevin's health. I actually understood the majority of what they were talking about when they were doing the overview. They did eye contact with me now and then and made sure that all of my questions are answered to the best of their knowledge.

Basically, this is what I was told. The work of the two organs, the kidneys and the lungs, that control his breathing and his blood pressure are currently being done by machine. Without the machine, he wouldn't last long at this point because his body wouldn't be strong enough to support itself. Test results are still pending to pinpoint information of the infection.

I am asking you to do a special dinner with your loved ones and pray together for Kevin and I tonight, okay?

Tuesday, August 3, 2010, 10:04 p.m.

Day 12, ICU 3, fifth e-mail

Joel and Mary Lou were the first to arrive at the hospital this morning. The doctors allowed us to have some time to pray over Kevin. We touched Kevin as we prayed. Joel and Mary Lou were denouncing the Devil and asked God to kill the illness and repair his organs. We prayed for comfort and strength to be restored. Kevin's temperature had lowered a little bit while we were in the room. I know this is due to prayer. Our God is so amazing!

We needed to give Kevin a break, so we went to the family waiting room to meet family members when they arrived. I told the medical staff that my kids and family were coming. They asked that we take turns being with Kevin. They felt that Kevin needed it as stress-free as possible right now.

After an hour or so had passed, Scott and my mother and father came along with the three kids. I went with the kids to see Kevin right away. We prayed together as a family. We also were able to have a moment of pause. During this time, I again touched Kevin and felt the warmth of his body. It was like I needed to remember this feeling of him alive more now than ever before. I didn't want to regret anything. I feared he was going to die this day.

After that, we went back to the waiting area and prayed with Joel and Mary Lou together as a family. They addressed the kids, and their individual fears. This time had allowed the kids to ask questions to Joel and Mary Lou to try to understand what was happening. They wondered why God didn't heal Kevin already when they have all asked him to. They are very concerned and scared. This was an awakening moment for the kids in their faith life. Each one of them felt better after this time with Joel and Mary Lou. They prayed out loud and gave Kevin, their dad, back to God and to the foot of the cross. After this, it's like they had a ton of bricks lifted from their shoulders. They weren't as afraid as when they first arrived and knew that they needed to trust that God was in charge no matter what the outcome would be.

Pastor Joel and Mary Lou made a *great* point today that might help anyone who is having a difficult time with this news so far. If we ask God to comfort us and give us peace, it will be much easier to deal with life's trials. Do we want to just sit there and be miserable? It is okay to be at peace with what is put in our paths as long as we give it to Jesus.

Before Joel and Mary Lou had left the hospital to go home, we were told that Kevin's kidneys had shown slight improvement. I was relieved, happy, confused, needing Kevin, and wanting this to be over. I do know that God heard our pleas and has proven his healing powers to us before. Remember all of the healing and miracles that has already happened during Kevin's illness? Remember the miracles at Abbott

Hospital? Where did the blood go? Where did the clot go that the doctors thought was in his heart and his brain?

The doctor's noticed a slight rash on Kevin's chest today. They thought that there might be a cell cluster in his chest to cause this. A cell cluster could have been caused from the stem cells growing too rapidly and clumped together. This is not a good situation for Kevin either. Just in case this is what is going on, the doctor's gave Kevin medicine that could possibly correct it if that's the case.

Kevin was put in a medicated coma so he has no pain and will not remember any of this. I am crushed that this is happening to us. Each one of us got to have a short amount of alone time with Kevin this morning. After a while longer at the hospital, we all went back to the Gift of Life House. I felt really bad for Stephanie. It is the rule of the Gift of Life House that no person under the age of seventeen is allowed past the first room of the house. The reason for this is that germs and sicknesses are carried by people under the age of seventeen more than those above the age of seventeen.

I wonder if she feels like an outcast. First of all, we told her she needed to leave her home and live with her dad. We thought this was the best thing to do for her. She can't stay with me or even truly visit in the gift house because of her age. I think she understands, but that might not make her feel any better. While I showed everyone else around the house, she needed to stay in the first room. It was nice and had a TV and couches, but I'm sure that she felt bad and alone. My sister, Penny, and sister-in-law, Brenda, arrived in the afternoon. We went to see Kevin and went out to lunch together. After lunch, we went back to the hospital to find that his temperature improved slightly.

Penny came prepared to stay overnight with me at the house. My appointment is early tomorrow, and it will be much better this way. I called the hospital at 9:50 p.m., and Kevin is still listed in critical condition. The doctor's were able to reduce the amount of blood pressure support. The ventilator is still helping Kevin to breathe, and he is comfortable.

I will update you all in the morning, as I feel you all need updates on the progress of Kevin. Remember to kiss your husband good night.

WEDNESDAY, AUGUST 4, 2010, 8:11 p.m.

Day 13, ICU 4

My sister, Penny, made me supper last night, gave me personal space, and supported me. I'm so glad that her main office for her job is down here in Rochester. Her boss was very nice to let her work down here for a couple of days.

My appointment was very stressful for me. The only paperwork that the doctor had received about my traumatic brain injury was the request for a second opinion that was sent by my specialist. The paperwork of test results, explanations, etc., was never received at the Mayo Clinic, Neurology Department. The doctor had the staff do some extra checking to see if they could locate them. Evidentially they were sent to a different office and couldn't get them to my appointment anymore.

When I found this out, I got very flustered and I had a difficult time focusing on what the doctor wanted. My sister, Penny, took a lot of notes and was a huge help for the doctor and me. My doctor had nothing to compare to, so she just asked me a ton of questions and did some simple tests.

Her decision was made. She wanted me to change my medication. She told me that my specialist back home has done exactly what he needed to and the Mayo can't do anything more than that. They can't help me. I instantly had a meltdown. I couldn't believe it! I was in so much pain and couldn't take it anymore. I was sick of the constant pain and headaches and pressure. I thought I was going to come down here and get a miracle treatment. Instead, I was told that I am not wanted as a patient here after this visit because I have a good doctor at home.

I don't really know if the doctor was surprised as to how I struggled with details or not, but the outcome was *not* what I was looking for at all. Being so very disappointed, I then realized that God *did* answer all of my requests. First of all, I asked for an appointment at the Mayo Clinic and I got it. I asked for good doctors with wisdom and I got it. I asked for something to help me and they changed my medications. I haven't had a recent MRI to send down to Rochester and I asked for one to be taken for their review. The doctor went out into the hallway and conferred with another doctor to see if this is what they wanted to do. They decided to schedule an MRI for me tomorrow. I asked for future news and I got it. I was told to continue my care in the cities and that I probably will have to live with this for the rest of my life.

I then needed to thank God for all of this even if it wasn't what I wanted. I was given the okay to work my old and new meds together for a little while and then wean off of my old one. This way, my aches wouldn't get unbearable like they usually would whenever I would switch medications.

After my doctor's appointment, Penny and I went to see Kevin. I was really sad for not having better news but again was glad it was over and that now we know that I need to live with this pain at the moment.

Kevin had a pretty good day today. He did have a fever of 101.5 this morning, but it was reduced with Tylenol. This high temperature, of course, came back later, but Kevin has been comfortable.

Kevin's urine has decreased quite a lot the last few days. The medical staff administered a drug called Lasix in hopes to help with that. The doctor's removed the blood pressure machine, and his pressure has been stable all day. They did another dose of the drug to help break up the extra stem cells in his chest as I explained in an earlier e-mail.

The test results for the infection still haven't come back. I was told that sometimes it can take up to a week for results to be completed.

They turned off the sedation that Kevin was receiving to try to clear his system of it. Kind of like giving his body a break from medicine. The sedation was replaced with the respirator during this time to help with his breathing. This lasted a little while until his agitation started to return. As soon as they saw this, they turned the sedation back on to keep him relaxed and comfortable.

Kevin is still listed in critical condition, and the doctors are on constant watch. I am very grateful for the much-needed support that we have received both here and at home. I've been singing a few times this week, which kind of helps me to pray and be comforted at the same time.

There are two songs that are really special to me. The words are perfect for how I feel about Kevin. After I sang the first song in the big atrium of the clinic, I noticed people had lined the railing on the second floor. They were listening in awe as if they could tell I was mourning. I also noticed others had stopped in their footsteps in front of me and were watching and listening. It was like they were respecting me and praying at the same time.

I typed the words for you to read. I sang the first one at our wedding.

He Has Chosen You for Me

We don't know what tomorrow holds, but we know who holds tomorrow.
Knowing this we'll live above the world and all its sorrows.
I have prayed for all my life that we would be together.
Serving him together seems so right.

Chorus:
Oh, oh yes, it's true.
He has chosen me for you.
Take my hand and we'll agree
That he has chosen you for me.

Now and then I like to think about the day he saved us.
All the love that he bestowed and all the gifts he gave me.
With all this I praise his name for putting us together.
He knew we'd be together from the start.

He has saved us.
Washed us white as snow
Now we're together
Cause he has made it so.

I have truly been blessed to have met and married Kevin. I am glad that Kevin is in my life but sad at the same time because he is in such pain and discomfort.

I Asked the Lord

I asked the Lord to comfort me, when things weren't going my way.
He said to me, "I will comfort you, and lift your cares away."
I asked the Lord to walk with me, when darkness was all that I knew.
He said to me, "Never be afraid, for I will see you through."

I didn't ask for riches, but he gave me wealth untold,
The moon, the stars, the sun, the sky, and he gave me eyes to behold.
I thank the Lord for everything, and I count my blessings each day,
For he came to me when I needed him, I only had to pray.

And he'll come to you if you ask him to.
For he's only a prayer away.

Some friends have called and expressed the need to see Kevin. They feel that if Kevin would die, they would need closure. They would need to see him yet while he was alive to tell him how they feel about him. They asked if they could come tomorrow or the day after to visit. I had told them that he isn't doing very well at this point. When I asked the medical staff if they were allowed to visit, they suggested that anyone who needs should come tomorrow.

Please don't forget why you love you husband or wife. Please let them know today because we don't know what tomorrow holds.

Talk with you tomorrow.

THURSDAY, AUGUST 5, 2010, 5:48 A.M.

Day 14, ICU 5

I don't sleep very well knowing that I'm not by Kevin. I called the ICU this morning at 4:15 a.m. and the nurse told me that there is no change from last night. I was relieved that it wasn't worse but sad that it wasn't any better either. The tests still show Kevin's kidney to be doing well at this time. This is good news for us.

I am concerned about Kevin's health. I asked for the kids to come down again today to spend some time here with him. I miss the kids also and feel the need for us all to be together.

Penny stayed overnight with me again last night so she could be available to come with me to my other doctor appointment today. The doctor appointment today will go over my MRI results from this morning. It was nice to have her here with me.

Yesterday, the doctors told me to call my specialist and go on the medication regimen that he suggests. When I called him, I understood him to say that I was to gradually go onto the new medication. Because my headaches are so bad, I still needed to stay on my current medication also.

When I went to see Kevin earlier today, before my MRI appointment, the neighbor's wife, in ICU, was crying because she thought her husband was dying. I definitely know now how she was feeling. She confided in me and was concerned, of course, about everything. They lived far away and have sold everything to be able to get here for medical help. I tried to be there for her for a short while. I hugged her, and we prayed together.

While we were praying, the ICU minister came over and had a visit with me. She told me that I wasn't to pray with this woman. It's personal for the family, and it's her job as a minister, not mine. I couldn't believe this! I was shocked, but respected her. I guess she probably wanted this woman to trust and rely on her.

I will update you on Kevin only if things change. It looks to be a busy day for me. Today is a new day. Let's not waste it! Love to you all!

THURSDAY, AUGUST 5, 2010

Day 14, ICU 5, second e-mail

When the kids arrived at the hospital, Penny and I were at my appointment. They called me and told me that Kevin opened his eyes and was responding to questions by winking his eyes or squeezing someone's finger when asked. Can you believe this? What a miracle! When Stephanie told me that his eyes opened, my heart felt like it was going to explode.

It was so nice to see Kevin and the kids together when we arrived to the room. We didn't want to visit for too long of a time because Kevin needed his rest. He has been through so much this week and has improved so much already. Kevin got really emotional when we were going to leave for lunch. I noticed this so I stayed with him.

Penny took the kids to the Gift House to make them lunch before she headed back to her home in Waconia. As Penny was on the way out of town, she dropped the kids back at the hospital for a short visit again before they headed for home.

I got a call in the early evening from our son, Tony. Tony was driving Kaylee's car, and evidentially, on the way home from Rochester, they got rear ended. He made sure to call me after the major stuff had already been handled.

Thank you, God, for watching out for them. The injuries were very minor. Kaylee had a sore neck and a headache, Tony's neck was stiff, and Steph had no injuries. The car was totaled out, but Tony told me that everything was fine. Kaylee had been checked over by the ambulance crew, and Tony and Steph didn't want to be checked out because they felt fine. My ex-husband, Tony and Stephanie's dad, picked the kids up and took them to the impound lot so they could get their personal stuff out of the car. Then he took them to our home in Howard Lake.

In the meantime, we will not mention anything about this to Kevin. He has enough on his plate right now, and we don't want him to get upset at all.

The nurses came in to put Kevin into a different bed. Once he was strapped in, they were able to arrange it and lift it to resemble a chair. Wow! Amazing! What an invention. I was told that this will be used for therapy to make Kevin stronger. They are hoping that this might also help relieve some of the excess fluid in his body. It was so nice to be able to talk with him while looking straight at him. He looked happy to be up and in the sitting position. What a change this was for both of us. I can't imagine how much better it must feel to be off of his back.

We haven't seen our friend, Rhonda, for probably ten years now. Kevin's illness has really been bothering her. She came for a visit tonight and had arrived in time to see Kevin while he was still sitting up. Kevin smiled and actually had a little sense of humor while visiting with her. It was like no time had passed since they last saw each other. It was so nice to hear the laughter and the snide comments given back and forth between the two of them.

Kevin got really tired after awhile being in this position. He was so weak yet and not able to hold his head up and support himself with his legs any longer. Rhonda offered to stay with Kevin while I went back to the house to shower and get stuff for spending the night with him. The funny thing about that was when Rhonda asked him if he wanted her to stay a while yet after I returned, he said "no". He wanted her to leave. She thought that was so funny. She said "It's just like Kevin to tell you like it is."

FRIDAY, AUGUST 6, 2010

Day 15, ICU 6

Kevin had a pretty good night last night and was fine when we woke up. I left the room to call home to check on the kids. I didn't want Kevin to overhear anything, even if he was slightly sedated. Tony told me that he had already taken care of the immediate insurance needs and had been in contact with Kevin's brother, Lester. We felt that the impound lot would deal better with an older adult than an eighteen-year-old. Lester was going to call the impound lot today to find out what was going on with the car and what needed to be done next in regard to the accident. I felt relieved at that time to know that someone was helping the kids with this matter and knew that I could figure everything else out on a different day.

We are fortunate to have my truck available for the kids to use if they needed to. Evidentially the whole back of the car, where Stephanie was sitting, was pushed all of the way into the passenger side backseat. Amazing how God's angels had their arms of protection around her. She didn't get even as much as a scratch on her. No headache, nothing other than a miracle.

After the call, I went to the bathroom to get cleaned up. When I returned to the room, the nurses were working on getting Kevin back up in the bed/chair like last night.

I was excited about that. I thought of it as another therapy session and a step forward. I enjoyed seeing him in the chair because he also didn't look as helpless. After a short while, it was clear to see that Kevin was getting tired and weak. He couldn't keep himself up in the chair anymore. His feet were slipping off of the footrest which in turn made him start to slip out of the chair. His legs were too weak to support himself.

I called the nurses and asked for help. They came in the room and resituated Kevin and asked him if he could wait just a few more minutes. They said that the doctor's were making their rounds, and they wanted to be ready for them. Kevin, of course, said, "Yeah, I can wait."

Soon after they left, he got weak again and couldn't keep himself up well at all. I tried to help him but knew that we needed the nurses to put him back in the bed. I called the nurses once again, and the same thing happened. They asked him to wait a few more minutes. He said "yes." As soon as they left, he asked me for help. I did the best I could and said, "That's good! Tell the nurses that you don't need them and as soon as they leave, you need help? I can't do this alone, and I don't want you to get hurt!"

I again called for the nurses and said, "Hey, he's weak and tired. I can't even keep his feet on the footrest." They said, "The doctors are almost here." Just at that time, the doctors came, and when they were done, the nurses put Kevin back. I was pissed! Why didn't I put my foot down? Why didn't I raise my voice to get it done? Why didn't I make them put him back in bed? Was I overcautious? I bet they deal with caregivers that are terrible from time to time very often. I guess I thought that they probably have done this many times before and had experience with this sort of thing. I didn't want to tell them how to do their job. I was focused and was able to handle it at the time. It was just really hard and concerning for me to see him struggle again.

Kevin's brothers, Wally and Paul, came to visit around 11:30 a.m. I met them outside and showed them where to park. As we were walking to the hospital, I informed them that Kevin isn't to know anything about the accident. It was really nice to see Kevin's eyes light up when his brothers walked into the room. Kevin got really excited. He wanted to talk but couldn't due to the respirator. This frustrated him.

They visited best they could for a few minutes, and then he got agitated. He was very upset and uncomfortable. It was a continuation of the morning chair episode. I don't know if it was a flare up or if the sedation had worn out at that time. I think that he was in the chair/bed too long this morning. Either way, he seemed upset, and I felt so bad for him. Remember, Kevin isn't fully sedated, just enough to keep him calm. They are trying to cleanse his body of this medication a little bit each day for as long as they can.

We all felt like Kevin needed some rest, so we told Kevin that we were going out to lunch and would be back soon. This was such a nice treat for me. During this lunch, it was like a break from the stress, even if it was just for an hour or so. When we had come back to the room, Kevin was still as agitated as when we had left. At this time, we don't even know if Kevin knew we were all there, so Paul and Wally went back home.

I had to leave the hospital for a while after his brothers left. I was having a very difficult time being in his room and watching him struggle again. Will this ever end? I was getting so frustrated. Rochester is such a nice town. There is an area between the Mayo buildings that is very calming. There is a small grass area with benches, specialty shops, coffee shops, and water fountains. I found a store that had great greeting cards. I enjoyed reading the humorous ones. It felt good to laugh.

After a few hours, I checked in on him and found him with a cold compress on his head. He had a fever of 101 degrees again and still had continued to be very restless. The medical staff increased his sedation medication from the previous dose in hopes that it would help. I always had brought work with me to do. I'm not a good person for just sitting there. I brought recipes that needed to be written on cards and filed. I brought thank you cards to write and I had a lot of time to read, write, and learn. A person can only do this stuff for so long, and they need to get out.

I felt comfortable with my surroundings as to where most everything is, so I was able to keep myself company and explore Rochester from time to time to get a break. I went to a bar across from the hospital to have a drink, and I had met an amazing young man there. I want to share his story with you.

He was blind and was in Rochester with his team for a blind baseball tournament this past week. It was amazing to hear as he explained to me how they play the game. The fielders and batters are blindfolded. The ball beeps and is a modified, and oversized, softball. The bases have electronics that cause it to buzz steadily when a switch is thrown. They are each placed 100 feet from home plate and are in the equivalent positions to first and third bases in regular baseball. When the batter hits the ball, a base operator turns on one of the two bases (first or third) for the batter to run to. If the batter touches the base before a fielder can pick up the ball, the offensive team scores a run. It takes 4 strikes for a batter to be out. This man was from Massachusetts and told me that he played seven games in four or five days. They played teams from all over the world. Isn't this amazing? This man has a handicap and you wouldn't even know it. He was having such a great time and talked as if this was nothing at all.

After my drink, I went back to Kevin's ICU room at around 8:00 p.m. and sat with him for a while. I always talked to him, even if I didn't know if he heard me or understood what I was saying. I planned my evening and decided that I needed to go to the house and get ready for the night at the hospital.

When I returned to the hospital, I had planned on relaxing and watching a movie. There was a TV in the hospital room, and it had free movie channels. The nursing staff told me that as long as Kevin doesn't get anxious, I can watch it quietly. I was so tired and had caught myself dozing off from time to time. I tried to sleep by his bedside for a while but felt like I was in the way.

The doctor's came into the room and did another chest x-ray and were working on Kevin's vitals and necessary treatments. Being as Kevin really didn't know if I was or wasn't there, I had decided that I needed to go to the Gift House again and try to get some sleep. I had difficulty sleeping because all I could think about was Kevin, knowing that the man I love is not here with me and replaying in my mind how I last saw him. I decided to get up and work on e-mails. I did, however, call to check up on him first and was told that he was having a good night but is still really sick and sedated.

SATURDAY, AUGUST 7, 2010, 7:45 A.M.

Day 16, ICU 7

Kevin had a slight fever again last night but it was manageable.

I talked to the nurse on the phone early this morning. They tried to reduce the sedation this morning but were unsuccessful. Kevin became very agitated again. I was concerned that they have not been able to manage or control his agitation yet. I explained what had happened at Abbott Hospital this past January when Kevin was agitated. I asked the nurse if it would be possible for them to check with Abbott to see what they did.

I know it's early, but I wanted to update you on some good news. Kevin's white cell count, fighting cells, is up from 0.1 to 0.5. The higher the count, the more cells there will be to help Kevin heal.

I want to extend my thanks for the prayers you have given for my grandma. Grandma is now out of the hospital and has returned back at her assisted living apartment in Norwood. She is getting checked on daily from the nurses, my parents and brother's and sister's families.

The car accident that the kids were involved in on Thursday night took a setback for Kaylee. She is really nervous to drive down here to visit Kevin today but feels the need to be here. I called our dear friends, Al and Dede, and explained the situation to them. They were more than happy to drive them all down for us.

I found out that no one was checking into or taking care of the car or anything regarding the accident anymore. I was really disappointed to find this out. I have decided that I needed to take charge and get this taken care of myself then. I contacted the impound lot and got the ball going. I've called a couple men I knew that deal with used cars to get the word out that I need to buy one for Kaylee to use. I've also started looking up the value of the car that was totaled so I can deal with the insurance company. I don't want them to take advantage of me and know that they will try because I'm a woman. I am fortunate to have a few people I can call for advice.

I will visit with you soon.

SATURDAY, AUGUST 7, 2010, 6:13 P.M.

Day 16, ICU 7, second e-mail

Kevin had a slight fever at times during the day today, but again, the medical staff was able to manage it.

Al and Dede brought Kaylee; her friend, Alex; and Stephanie down today and were happy to see Kevin open his eyes. He knew they all were here, but we needed to leave because he got too agitated again. I imagine that he wanted to talk and let us know he is all right. That's the kind of man he is.

Before Kevin had been sedated, I told him I wanted to shave my head to support him. He didn't want me to. He said, "Why do I want to look at a bald wife?" You know how some people wear bracelets to remind them to do something? Example, WWJD bracelets remind you to pray. Well, I decided to buy scarves to wear instead of shaving my head. My hair is covered, and it is a support reminder for me and everyone to pray for sick people.

I asked the girls if they would wear scarves on their head to support Kevin. They, of course, were excited about this, so we went to a store that carried beautiful scarves that women from India wear. They were inexpensive and beautiful. Once the girls picked out a couple of them, we went to lunch for some quality time.

On the way to lunch, I noticed two men walking with sticks due to blindness. They must have been in town for the baseball tournament also. Everyone but Stephanie had already walked into the restaurant. These two men were definitely happy to be here and trusted their own direction. They seemed to not have a care in the world. I don't know why, but for some reason, I had the feeling that they were going the wrong way. I stopped them and asked them where their destination was. At that moment, I had the most wonderful feeling come over me as I was able to tell them the correct way to go. I put their arm around mine to turn them to the right direction. I wasn't going that way, so I asked some men to please finish taking them where they needed to go.

After lunch, we went back to see Kevin. We took turns visiting with him and he seemed fine with short visits.

Kevin hasn't been having any bowel movements for a few days now. The doctors decided to have the liquid food cut until they figure out why this is happening. They took an x-ray of his stomach in hopes to get an answer. I don't know if they gave him an enema or not but the nurse just came in and told me that there just was a tiny bowel movement. It is important that they find out if there is a blockage. Whatever the reason is, they need to find it. They don't want it to interfere with his breathing. Can you imagine? What next?

They are still waiting for test results to see if Kevin has an infection or not. In the meantime, they are still treating him with a broad-range antibiotic just in case.

The following is what was discussed during the doctor's rounds this morning: There is going to be a consultation on Monday to see if Kevin needs to have a tracheotomy. I will be very pleased if he gets this. I feel Kevin would deal with the tracheotomy better than having this tube down his throat. I feel it would be less stressful for him. They also talked about the original central line that was put in Kevin for the collection of cells. It's already been in for one month. I'm wondering if they will take that one out. I don't know at this time but am concerned.

I don't know how Kevin is truly feeling right now. I feel he has been steadily getting weaker since yesterday. We need to take one day at a time and keep our prayers going.

I try to be by Kevin as much as I can because I feel he needs me by his side. I hold his hand, touch his face, and talk to him. His hair is falling out quite a bit now. I have been able to pull some out, but now it's getting all over the pillows. I don't like this because I think it's unclean. I asked the nurses to shave his head for this reason. It's going to come out anyway, so just get it over with.

I'll e-mail soon. Thanks!

SATURDAY, AUGUST 7, 2010, 10:44 P.M.

Karen talk, third e-mail

I wanted to take a break from the ICU room. Kevin's not here to talk to, so I'm organizing and want to e-mail some information to you all before I put it away. I found information from the Mayo Clinic on soap versus sanitizer comparison that I want to share with you all. This is word for word on their pamphlet.

First, you need to remove visible contamination/dirt with soap and water. You shouldn't have the sanitizer do this. After the visible dirt is gone, use waterless alcohol-based hand rubs. These hand rubs come in the form of a gel or foam and usually can be purchased wherever hand soap is sold. Hand cleaning with an alcohol-based hand rub is faster than using soap and water and may cause less skin irritation and dryness.

In addition, it is as effective as soap and water when hands are not visibly soiled. Antibacterial soaps contain agents that may cause organisms to become resistant and more difficult to kill. For this reason, we don't recommend their use in the home. Alcohol-based hand rubs kill bacteria without making them resistant. This makes hand rubs okay for use in all places whenever our hands are not visibly soiled. If you have any questions about this, call the Mayo Clinic and ask to speak to someone from Infection Prevention and Control 507-284-2511.

I also met and visited with a young woman from Israel. She told me that she lives on a man-made island. It is beautiful there and a really nice place to live. She said that it's kind of like Las Vegas and New York.

I asked her why women have to wear so many clothes and the men can wear short-sleeved shirts when it is so hot. I understood her explanation. It is tradition and just the way it is. I still thought that the men should have to cover up and wear more clothes too.

This young lady showed me some tricks. She pulled up her sleeve and showed me that it looks like she has another long-sleeved shirt underneath the cloth, but it's just a long glove. She told me that the material is very comfortable, and they are used to it being hot. They can wear anything they want underneath the cover and don't need to dress like this until the family thinks that she has gone through puberty. This is usually at the age of fifteen or sixteen years old. She laughed and said that sometimes she even goes out in her pajamas and nobody knows because she's covered up. At home, they can go without the sheets when only relatives are around.

Diana is a young woman from Waverly who is very active in working for Christ. She is active in the youth group in our church back home in Howard Lake when she's home. I didn't know this, but Diana currently lives down here in Rochester. She just came back from a mission trip in Gowanda and called to ask if I needed anything. At that time, I just wanted to be alone. I didn't feel like talking or doing anything with anyone. She offered to pick me up and take me to church with her tomorrow morning at 9:15 a.m. I thought that I might feel differently tomorrow, so I accepted her invitation.

I'm starting my new medication tonight that the Mayo doctor recommended. I sure hope this one helps me.

I just got really sleepy now, so I have to go. Take care and sending a lot of hugs.

SUNDAY, AUGUST 8, 2010, 6:45 A.M.

Day 17, ICU 8, first e-mail

I wanted to see Kevin before church today, so I came in early to spend some time with him. The nurse wanted Kevin to be very still and quiet, so the lights were turned off, there were no sounds in the room, and I just sat by him holding his hand and feeling his pulse. I don't want to regret anything!

Kevin had a pretty good night. His temperature stayed normal, but his blood pressure was a little low. He did have bowel movements and this should make him feel more comfortable. The nurse told me that a lot of times, the medication will clog your system, which creates gas. I was told that the results from the test yesterday on his stomach have not come back yet. He just had another bath and is resting comfortably, so I decided that now would be a good time for an e-mail update.

This morning, I was irritated at the nurses. I have been watching them all so very closely while they are working on or with Kevin during this hospital stay. Each nurse does things a little different. These particular nurses didn't have support for the bottom of Kevin's feet like I wanted or felt he needed; the respirator wasn't supported under his chin, which made it push down on his lower lip. This looked so uncomfortable. They turned Kevin, supporting him on one side. Then they put pillows under both legs. This made his body and spine uneven. I wanted a pillow under one leg so he would be comfortable.

I put pillows at the foot of the bed to give support for Kevin's feet. He needs his toes to point up to keep his muscles strong. I asked them to fix the respirator and the pillows for his legs. After all of this, the nurse asked me when the last time was when he was sitting up in the chair. I sternly told them, "No, he was up too long on Friday, and the doctors said he wasn't ready for this right now." I told her that she needed to ask the doctor first before doing this again. By the way, these were the same nurses that left him up too long Friday morning and didn't listen when I asked for them to put him back in bed.

I was so frustrated! My brain isn't working right now. I can't even think of what I do to get myself going right now. I don't know what to do. Maybe someone here needs somebody to talk to. Well, I saw the ICU neighbor that I prayed with last week. She came up to me and hugged me so hard for being there for her. Each time we see each other we hug and give a warm smile. It helps each one of us. She told me today that her husband is doing fine at the moment. I was so thankful for answered prayers once again.

I feel the need to do something that's normal for a change. It didn't take long to find something. Someone left the coffee pot on the burner when it was empty at the hospital, so I cleaned it up. When I got back to the Gift House to get ready for church, I had noticed that there were dishes that needed to be run through the sanitizer.

If you look, there is always something to do to help anywhere and anytime.

Today is another day to decide if we are going to live it in fullness or sit back and feel lazy or sorry for ourselves.

Have a great day. I'll e-mail later.

SUNDAY, AUGUST 8, 2010, 4:09 P.M.

Day 17, ICU 8, second e-mail

I need prayers for myself and Kevin. I've lost hope! I don't know what happened, where it went, and what to do! Maybe it's because I'm really tired, I started my new pills last night, or maybe I'm just not doing something right. I've been trying so hard to stay positive and have a good attitude for my kids and family, but I don't have the feeling that things are getting much better. I have total peace and guess I feel guilty that I have resided to the fact that all I can do is just continue to pray and not worry. Right now, I'm at such peace that I feel like I'm going to be okay if Kevin doesn't make it. I feel guilty feeling that way. It's like I don't want him to be struggling anymore and I will let him go if God wants him.

Diane had overslept and called to inform me that she won't make it to church with me. I went to church anyway this morning. Believe me I tried to find any reason not to go. I wanted to come up with anything in order to make me feel like I shouldn't or couldn't go. Reasons like Diane overslept so she can't go with me; I was tired; if one of the two churches I walk to doesn't start at 9:30, I'm not going; if I can't take communion because I'm not that religion, I'm not staying; etc. Well, there wasn't communion today, and the second church I walked to actually did start at 9:30.

I don't know if I got anything out of the sermon message or not, but I did pray. I really don't feel any different now than before I went to church. I just feel helpless. Don't get me wrong, I don't need company. I'm not lonely either. I'm just doing my thing when I want and what I want. I just need to be alone and be with Kevin every chance I get.

Jim and Kim came for a visit in the early afternoon today. They are very good friends of ours. Kevin had been friends with them for many years before we were married. They all have gone on snowmobiling trips together, been on a racquetball team, and a baseball team together for many years. Jim and Kim both are so much fun to be around. They are always lighthearted and full of laughter. When Kevin and I got married and we all started getting busy with our kids, we saw less and less of each other but still have a bond that nobody could ever break.

I saw the hurt in their eyes as we sat in the waiting room and I explained Kevin's situation personally to them. I was already feeling helpless, and they could sense that.

When we went in to see Kevin, they enjoyed reading the "get to know me" poster that I had made, explaining things about Kevin like what's his favorite show; things that stress me out, which I answered "not being with my wife"; achievements; things that cheer me up; etc. They needed to add a few things to the poster and enjoyed being a part of it. It was plain to see how hard it was for them to leave Kevin but still were glad to have spent this time here with him.

In the afternoon, I had a phone call from one of the kids. There was a problem at home. Everyone was afraid that they were doing more work than the others. I tried to help them solve the problem but had no success. I was already stressed with Kevin and tried to explain to them that I didn't need to deal with this right now. Our phone conversation had ended unsettled. I wasn't home to control or help with the situation, so I called our friend, Greg. I told him that I respected his work value and discipline morals. I had asked him to please go over to the farm and settle this issue. I was relieved and sure that this situation at home would be taken care of instantly. The kids weren't happy at all about sending Greg over, but the work got done.

Today is another day to decide if we are going to live it in fullness or sit back and feel lazy or sorry for ourselves.

SUNDAY, AUGUST 8, 2010, 8:53 P.M.

Day 17, ICU 8, third e-mail

I'm stumped maybe because I'm tired. I don't know; I can't even think of the future without Kevin. I made a list of things that I'm looking forward to experiencing with him. I have read these off out loud at one of my visits in his room. I'm hoping that he can hear me and comprehend what I said. We have so much fun together, and I don't want to plan any of these things without him:

Tony coming home to visit from college
Tony maturing after he's been at college for a little while
Stephanie appreciating home more
Kaylee's volleyball and softball games
Holiday parties at our home
Our children's graduation parties
Weddings
Grandchildren
Dogs

Basketball
Snowshoeing
football games
Friends

MONDAY, AUGUST 9, 2010, 3:46 A.M.

Day 18, ICU 9, Just a few words

Here's what I was looking for yesterday, but I got frustrated and quit. I hope this helps everyone in their time of need or trials in whatever is presently going on in your life like it is mine.

Karen: After speaking with you on the phone this morning I went to my Bible and I wanted to find you some comforting quotes that I feel could put some comfort at this time of unknown.

"Listen, Lord, to my cries for help. I call to you in times of trouble, because you answer my prayers." (Psalm 86:6, 7)

"Keep on asking and you will be given what you ask for. Keep on looking and you will find. Keep on knocking and the door will be opened." (Matthew 7:7)

I am a firm believer that God has messages for us through his words. I am sure that there have many times over the past several months and even days that you have felt frustration but then I want you to read this quote from the Bible to yourself. You will be constantly reminded that God's timing is NOT ours and his plan is NOT ours.

Psalm 33:20 says, "We wait in hope for the Lord; he is our help and our shield."

That's what you need to do, Karen. Wait and TRUST that the Lord will reveal HIS plan to you, Kevin, and the doctor's in HIS time.

"We can make our plans, but the Lord determines our steps." (Proverbs 16:9)

Well, that just sums it all up. It doesn't matter when, what, or how many plans we make for ourselves, the Lord will determine the steps that we take and when we take them.

Love you all,

Rhonda
Ps. I hope that these quotes help and bring you some peace in your heart.

I printed off each of these verses and taped them to the poster of Kevin. They will be in plain sight for us to read out loud to him from time to time. These words will uplift both Kevin and the reader.

MONDAY, AUGUST 9, 2010

Day 18, ICU 9

This morning, when the kidney doctor came in, he asked the night nurse if they have been giving Kevin something. I can't remember but think it was water because of his high sodium levels. The nurse said, "No, we didn't." The doctor looked very disappointed and that upset me.

Kevin's family, Nancy, John, and Lester came to visit and took me out to lunch to spoil me. I told them all that had happened and how upset I was. My in-laws thought that possibly, I just needed to relax and let the nurses do what they need. They told me that the nurses went to school for this and are highly educated. I need to relax and get away from here. Maybe they are right. I need some time away.

After lunch, we all came back to see Kevin again. Lester, John, and Nancy were able to hold Kevin's hand and talk to him briefly before they went back home.

In the afternoon, Konnie, who is the wife of Kevin's childhood friend and neighbor, had called. Her husband and she have been keeping up on the news of Kevin via my e-mail updates. She just so happened to be in Rochester for work today for meetings and training. Konnie and I have met each other about two or three times before today and really didn't know each other very well. She wanted to get together for the evening for dinner and time out. We connected and really enjoyed each other's company right away.

The time flew so fast, and it was so much fun. We, of course, didn't have any problem talking, meeting others, and visiting. It made me forget for a while why I was in Rochester. She was a positive influence for me today and had told me not to look at the future as far as Kevin getting more transplants but to concentrate on Kevin getting better right now.

TUESDAY, AUGUST 10, 2010, 8:48 A.M.

Day 19, ICU 10, first e-mail

Not much has happened since the last e-mail, other than ups and downs for both Kevin and me. For the most part, Kevin needs his rest and his breathing regulated. His kidneys seem to be working much better now, which is really good. The specialist said we need to take it one day at a time. There are still cultures from the lung tests that haven't been completed yet. The ones that have been completed are negative for infection. I will find out today if his stomach is absorbing food yet.

Kevin has a lot of fluid buildup, and the doctor's are working on that also. Over the night, the doctors were a little concerned because Kevin had a temperature of 99 degrees, which isn't bad at all but something that needs to be watched. His breathing was also fluctuating. They added a different medicine to see if this would calm him down more, and it seemed to work. I called a number of times throughout the night to check on him. It's hard to sleep because I'm not by his side. Each time, it was reported back to me that he was resting well.

My hope has improved a little bit, but I still need help with that. I think the kids are in denial, even though they know he is really sick. My sister, Vicki, and my parents are visiting today.

The assistant youth director at our church, Jen, was in town visiting her aunt today. Her aunt is a hospital nursing supervisor at the Mayo hospitals. They are both stopping in to see Kevin and me.

I will e-mail again soon.

Tuesday, August 10, 2010, 10:19 a.m.

Day 19, ICU 10, second e-mail

The ICU doctors just came by and visited with me.

Kevin is still really sick, but his kidneys and blood pressure are better. Kevin is also really swollen. The doctors are concerned and know the necessity of getting the excess fluids out of Kevin's body. Once they succeed in reducing the fluids, they feel it will also help with his breathing.

Wednesday, August 11, 2010, 10:02 a.m.

Day 20, ICU 11, first e-mail

Kevin was *very angry* this morning in bed when the sedation was reduced and had been thrashing around ever since because he is frustrated. The thing is, he doesn't even know it. He won't remember any of this and doesn't know what he is doing.

It's been hard for me to watch him the last few days because I can't do anything. I mean in January, my job was to keep him calmed down and in bed. If I couldn't handle him, my job was to call for help. Here, I can't help. He can't even get out of bed if he'd want to, but needs to heal inside. I'm helpless for him, but I do understand it.

Today seems to be a pretty good day so far. I will stay around here for a while this morning just to see if I'm needed for the transition, but then I will leave. The doctor's know what they are doing, and I don't have to be here.

This is another long e-mail. I feel this is necessary to type in detail so everyone understands. I feel I need to explain why Kevin has so much excess fluid. It's easier for me to understand if it's explained in great detail and then write it down so I can refer back to it, if I forget. I feel it's good for you also to hear from me as to what's happening to Kevin here and that it's written the same for everyone to read. This will eliminate gossip. Let me know if you have any questions or don't understand and I will help.

First of all, Kevin's cells were put back in his system during his transplant. This happened on day 0, which was 20 days ago. The cells started to engraft. Engraftment is when the cells start taking their proper place in the system. Kevin's cells were engrafting faster than anyone had expected. This is called peri engraftment syndrome and can cause a lot of problems. The peri engraftment may have allowed chemicals to cause Kevin's vessels to leak fluid. When this happens, the fluid goes to other parts of the body like the lungs. This would cause breathing difficulties also.

Kevin's blood pressure became high, which could cause damage to the organs. Kevin's kidneys were affected by this, so they weren't operating as they should. This means that they weren't able to get rid of fluid like they needed to. The fluid just kept building up, and as of yesterday, Kevin was carrying thirty-five extra pounds of fluid alone in his system. His ears had been puffy and his ankles, knees, neck, wrists, and legs were huge. Dialysis could help with this problem, but the doctor's really don't want to do this unless they have to. If they decide to do dialysis, it could cause infection to set in. They felt it would be beneficial to wait for a few days to see if his kidneys improve and do the work of releasing fluids by themselves. It's amazing how our body was created isn't it?

When the kidney's work and the fluids are drained from the vessels, the excess fluid that's in the other parts of Kevin's body will get sucked back into his vessels. It all works together.

Remember when I told you about the cell collection and how the medicine Kevin was given caused excess stem cells to be made in the bone marrow? When there was no more room in the bone marrow to house them, they would go into the vessels for collection. Well, this is the opposite. The vessels need fluid. When drained, they will get the excess fluid back and continue until the proper amount is left. In order for that to happen, the organs need to work. His lungs should also improve with removal of the excess fluid that's in them.

Kevin's stomach isn't absorbing quite enough food, but his bowel movements are finally working pretty well, so the doctor's aren't worried about this at this time. Kevin's lung test results showed *no* infection, but this doesn't necessarily mean that there is none. The doctors told me that sometimes it just doesn't show up on the culture slide but really is there. In all, Kevin has seen improvement in the last twenty-four hours.

We are all hoping and praying that Kevin will accept the transition of the breathing respirator so he can relax and heal better.

WEDNESDAY, AUGUST 11, 2010

Day 20, ICU 11, second e-mail

I don't know how they did it, but the doctors were able to remove the respirator. Who cares at this point how they did it. The fact of it being out is wonderful news for all of us. Once the respirator was out, Kevin could communicate a little bit. His throat was really rough, and he had a difficult time talking. He still continued to be agitated because he still couldn't get out of bed.

He was much angrier at me because I wouldn't and/or couldn't help him. Example, you know how some people can look at you with such anger that it just shoots right through you? Well, this is the look I got from Kevin. At times, when I was holding his hand, he would dig his fingernails into my hand so hard that it felt like I was bleeding. He didn't draw blood, but I did have marks.

Later on, my sister, Penny, and her husband, Alan, brought Kaylee and Stephanie down here. As we were all visiting with Kevin, he was talking to us and calling us dumb asses all of the time. Some thought it was funny and laughed because it sounded just like him, but I was actually deeply hurt. Now we all know that Kevin really isn't angry like this. This was caused by his coming off all of those drugs. He doesn't even remember any of this ever happened.

Later on that day, I was angry, not at God, not at Kevin, but at the situation. I felt like saying, "Come on, let's get it over with already. Why are you punishing us? What do you want me to do?"

THURSDAY, AUGUST 12, 2010, 4:43 A.M.

Day 21, ICU 12

Thank you for all your prayers! Kevin had a turnaround in the last twenty-four hours. I pray that it stays.

Kevin has been breathing well with the use of an oxygen mask. This also gives his throat the much-needed moisture so his throat will heal from the tube.

At the doctors' rounds this morning, I will find out more. I will ask if the excess fluid is still of concern, if the kidneys are working to their capacity, and if the stomach has improved.

I have called a number of times throughout the night. One time, the nurse said they were asking Kevin where he was and what had happened to him. Kevin evidently did so well that today, he was moved out of the ICU to the regular floor. This is so exciting. Everything that has already gone on. One moment, he is dying, and the next moment, he is healing better than expected. The doctor's were right with their tactics. Kevin's blood pressure and kidneys started working as they needed, which in turn cleaned out his body of excess fluids. What a miracle again!

I was excited about this and got a boost of energy to do something. Kevin needed to rest anyway, so I went back to Jo-Ann Fabric and got more material to make more do-rags. This time, I got fun prints. Vikings, camouflage, peace signs, wildlife, etc. I decided that I was going to sew them and donate them to the cancer house.

As I was walking back to the hospital from the transplant house, I stopped and asked a couple of young ladies, who seemed to be students, about the building they were waiting to get into. All I wanted to know was some history of it. One of the ladies had their mother with her. The mom got mad at me because I talked to her daughter. She moved toward me and said, "Please step back. I don't want you near my daughter. Leave! Go away from us!" I said, "I only am trying to ask a question. I'm not going to do anything." She just got closer to me and said, "Go now!" I mean, come-on! What in the world is this country girl going to do? All I wanted was to be nice to others and converse.

The doctors and nurses on the ICU floor had firsthand exposure to this miracle of life that occurred with Kevin. They were so amazed. I'm sure that they can testify many miracles in their line of work.

When Kevin got to his regular hospital room, the medical staff there too was sure of the miracle that occurred with Kevin. Not only there but also at the Gift House, and my e-mail update readers were made aware of this wonderful news and second chance at life.

Last night, Kevin threw up quite a bit. The doctor's were concerned slightly about this. I have no idea why this happened.

Take care and praise the Lord of all!

FRIDAY, AUGUST 13, 2010

Day 22, hospital 1

Kevin stopped puking today.

My friends, Mary and Patti, came to Rochester to visit us tonight. Mary surprised us when they arrived. She had shaved her head a couple of days ago to support Kevin. She looks great! They planned on staying overnight at the hotel next to the hospital so we can have a girls' night and I won't have to be that far away from Kevin. I miss them so much.

Mary told me that there were so many people back home who have asked for a Caringbridge Web site to be created. There are a couple of reasons that she felt this would be helpful. First of all, there are some who want to know what's going on with Kevin and aren't on the e-mail list that I have been sending. Secondly, there are some that only want to read the facts and not my thoughts, feelings, or religious beliefs. I told her to go ahead and do it, but I don't want to be responsible for keeping it up. She gladly took that job upon herself. What a friend.

Have a great weekend.

SATURDAY, AUGUST 14, 2010

Day 23, hospital 2

I truly feel guilty that I had so much fun last night. I mean, Kevin is here lying in the hospital and I left him to go out with my friends.

Our friends, Greg and Nancy, came down to see us in the afternoon today. We had a nice long visit, and when Kevin needed to rest, I was able to show them around the town a little bit. This was very relaxing for me, and Kevin really enjoyed visiting with them also.

SUNDAY, AUGUST 15, 2010

Day 24, hospital 3

I decided not to listen to Kevin for the first time in my life. I got my head shaved this morning. I went to the nurses' station and asked for one of them to shave it down to the scalp. They were so surprised, excited, and cautious. The nurse I chose told me that she isn't used to cutting off such long hair, but she would do the best she could. It felt really weird, but I was determined to do this to support Kevin.

After my hair was off, I instantly went to see Kevin. When I walked into the room, Kevin looked at me and started to cry. I told him that I know he doesn't want to lose his hair and now we can grow our hair back together. Kevin was thankful and proud of this support.

Tonight, the doctors pulled Kevin's catheter for his urine output. Shortly after that, Kevin started having sensations of needing to urinate every five to fifteen minutes. When the sensations came on, he'd call for me, and I would need to help him. There was more blood with the urine at first, but the nurses told us that this is normal due to the catheter irritation. This continued *all* night. The blood did lessen as the night went on. Put it this way, we didn't get much sleep at all.

MONDAY, AUGUST 16, 2010

Day 25, hospital 4

Well, I did it! I got all of the necessary information put together to present it to the insurance company for reimbursement of the car. I did a really good job too and was very pleased with my accomplishment.

Kevin didn't feel well at all today! He even called me over to the bed and just held my hand. He looked really scared.

When the doctors came in, they ordered an ultrasound of his stomach. The results showed that Kevin had over 900ml of urine in his bladder. The amount usually required before they would consider insertion of a catheter is 400ml. I can't even begin to imagine how much pain he was in!

The doctors reinserted the catheter in the evening to drain the urine. It was explained to us that sometimes, when the catheter is used for a long period of a time, the bladder may stop working. It needs to be retrained to work properly.

I thought instantly, *Oh, my God! Now the bladder has stopped working?* The doctors assured me that they would take care of this and make Kevin comfortable once again.

I felt the need of being alone and relaxing. I wanted to just escape and forget that I was here for just a little while. I went to listen to the Rochester Carillon perform its normal Monday evening concert at 7:00 p.m. The Carillon music can be heard for blocks away. I decided to lie on the grass right under the bell tower where the music comes out of in the Annenberg Plaza. I was disappointed that the music wasn't clear but didn't realize that it all depended on the weather and is usually heard better a few blocks downwind.

As I was resting peacefully. I was so relaxed and didn't care what others thought of me lying on the grass in the middle of the park. I saw a number of dogs around and really missed and longed to hug and pet one. For some reason, I was in need of unconditional love from an animal. All of a sudden, I noticed an elderly woman leading the cutest little dog. I had a great desire to hug, pet, and hold this little creature. I prayed for them to come my way, so I could stop them and fulfill my need.

Wouldn't you know it? All of a sudden, the dog got away from its owner. I saw it and was hoping so hard that it would run to me. Guess what? It did! I couldn't believe this! All of the people and open space around, and he came to me! Evidentially, the woman's sick husband was twenty feet the other direction from me, but the dog still came right to me. The owner came and retrieved him as fast as she could. I reassured her of how much I needed that dog at that particular moment. She introduced me to her husband, and they explained to me of his sickness. They came to the Mayo Clinic in hopes for a miracle for his skin disease. We enjoyed each other's company for quite some time and helped each other get lifted up.

TUESDAY, AUGUST 17, 2010, 4:49 P.M.

Day 26, hospital 5

This morning, the catheters for the urine and stool were removed for a test trial of six hours. They will replace them again only if they need to drain excess urine. They will repeat the process every six hours, until the bladder and prostrate learn to work again.

Kevin just got done with another therapy session and has improved greatly in his strength.

I thought it would be nice for Kevin to see what he looks like with no hair. So I took a picture of both of us.

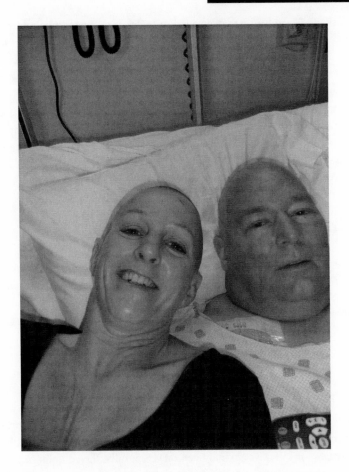

We were just visited by my friend, Ardella, and her daughter-in-law. They were pleasantly surprised at Kevin's attitude and how well he looks.

I haven't e-mailed much lately because I wasn't comfortable sharing everything that was happening to us at the time. Last week, I had lost my hope and desire to keep begging God for a miracle. I actually got to the point as to accept Kevin's death, being at peace with it and knowing that we will all be all right without him. I knew it would be tough, but it would be easier to just have this done and over with and not see Kevin go through any more misery or pain.

He was so very sick, and when the doctor's would tell me good news like "The blood pressure machine is now shut off, and Kevin's doing this on his own now" or "His kidneys are still doing at least some of the work," I felt a kind of relief, but when I asked them, "So he isn't in critical condition anymore right?!" their reply was, "Oh, yes, he is a very sick man and in very critical condition." I was confused as to what to think of these comments, especially when they are given to me daily.

As these mixed feelings continued, I felt ashamed because I gave up my part of the fight.

As the doctor's reduced Kevin's sedation to see if that would help him relax and improve his health, Kevin became very agitated and made it harder for him to breathe. He is going through so much, and I couldn't stand to watch it anymore. I then felt like I was being selfish because things weren't going my way, so I decided to stay away from the hospital a little more while Kevin is being weaned of the sedation.

After some alone time, I noticed that I just didn't feel anything anymore. I was sad, empty, confused, sorry, and irritated. I wasn't lonely because I have so many people I could call, but how do you explain this? One of the days that I went to the transplant house (where we are staying) to do laundry, I talked to a mother who has a very sick daughter and shared my feelings with her in shame. She understood to the point that she told me that she feels like that a lot also. She actually seemed to be relieved to be able to talk about this to someone. That's one of the reasons I wanted to share all of this personal info. Maybe there is someone we don't know who reads this that is in the same place.

God bless you and yours, and please continue the prayers because remember, I gave up the fight and didn't ask anymore and notice the miracle? You all were praying! Thank you and thank you, God!

WEDNESDAY, AUGUST 18, 2010, 2:57 P.M.

Day 27, hospital 6

Kevin had a good night last night and his bladder is finally working on its own. We are both very relieved. His hemoglobin is a little low yet. Kevin's white grafting cell count has decreased the last two days, but the doctor's are thinking that it's because of all of the medications that Kevin had been on. Hopefully, the cell numbers will come back up. Kevin's potassium level was low today, so he had to have an IV to bring this back up. All of this doesn't sound perfect, but he is sound enough to get transferred to St. Mary's Rehab Center in Rochester tomorrow morning for more intense therapy.

At first when we heard of this move, I was very concerned. Are they going to take good enough care of him? Will they be able to keep up on his vitals? Later on, I found out that St. Mary's is an inpatient center just like a hospital. They will do blood tests, give proper medications at the correct times, check all of his vitals, and everything that Methodist does for Kevin. He still needs to be somewhere that's close to the hospital and needs extra therapy, so we agreed that this is the right place to be.

Kevin will have therapy an average of three hours every day. Therapy will include both physical and occupational therapies. I will continue to reside at the transplant house and sleep at night at the rehab facility. There is a washing machine for me to use there for ease of washing Kevin's clothing, etc. I will have the opportunity to get away and take time for myself while Kevin is in therapy. The rehab facility is close to the transplant house and I can walk back and forth. This will give me time to sew my do-rags and make my meals. Kevin's meals will be served at 8:00 a.m., noon, and 6:00 p.m. This is really scheduled so it's easier to plan therapy schedules for the patients.

We are very excited for this step forward, and I will keep you updated.

Sanitation is still very important at this time for Kevin. He will need to have a private room to reduce the spread of germs. Everyone who enters this room will need to wash their hands before they enter and after they leave. Nobody is allowed if they have any kind of illness or cold. After all that has happened, we don't need Kevin to get sick or an infection.

I personally feel that Kevin's body still needs healing but know that he's on the right track. Thank you for all of your wonderful prayers and words of encouragement.

Chapter 10

Rehab and Set Backs

Thursday, August 19, 2010, 6:28 p.m.

Day 28, Kevin's rehab 1

Today, around one o'clock, Kevin arrived at St. Mary's Rehab. He would have been there sooner in the day, but the hospital wanted him to have a bag of red blood cells and one bag of fluids administered before he left. This is due to his hemoglobin being low again today.

We were both so excited to have our son, Tony, visit in the morning and be there for the move to St. Mary's. Kevin was transported by the Gold Cross ambulance because that was the only safe way for him to be moved at this time. I'm glad Tony was able to go in the ambulance with Kevin. He probably didn't appreciate it like I thought he would, but I wanted both of them to experience this part of Kevin's move together.

Once I figured out where the underground parking was and got up to the room, Kevin and Tony were already there. Tony waited and got the Internet going on our laptop computer so we could use it during our stay here. Tony and I were taken on a short tour of the rehab facility. This is truly an amazing place with its beauty and history.

When we got back to Kevin's room, we presented Tony with his college gift from the two of us. I wanted Kevin to be a part of this because this is such a big step for Tony. We are both so very proud of him.

When Tony left, Kevin and he just shook hands. No hug or kiss like I always need, but a firm handshake.

Kevin was visited by doctors the rest of the day until 5:00 p.m. They were testing him and getting to know his strengths and weaknesses. This will help in the determination of the therapy schedules that are necessary. Once the treatment is decided, Kevin will get his ongoing therapy schedules for the next day around 6:00 p.m. the night before. This schedule will include both occupational and physical therapy sessions.

Kevin's spirits are wonderful, and I feel better knowing that Kevin's vitals will be taken one time a day and the doctors at the Mayo Clinic and the Eisenberg Hospital will be kept informed of Kevin's ongoing health conditions. When Kevin is strong enough to be released from St. Mary's rehab, we will still need to get approval to come home from the Mayo Clinic.

We are still in need of your wonderful prayers. Notice the miracle that occurred again!?

FRIDAY, AUGUST 20, 2010

Day 29, rehab 2

This morning, I needed to come home to do some much-needed yard work and move our son, Tony, to North Dakota State University for college. I had mixed emotions. I was sad to leave Kevin alone, happy for Kevin's health improvement, sad for Tony to go to college, but happy for this new chapter in his life also.

Kevin understood the reason that I couldn't stay with him for the weekend, but at the same time, he was very sad. He doesn't like to be alone down here at all. He was concerned about all of the driving I would be doing. We decided that I would not come back until Sunday. This would give me a break from driving and get some rest.

Before I left Rochester, I called Kevin's brother, Lester, and asked him and his wife, Sharon to come down the next day to visit with Kevin. I knew that I would feel better leaving if he had some company. If nothing else, it certainly will help pass the time away for Kevin.

I told Stephanie that I wanted her to move back home this past week. I needed her to have some time with Tony before he left for college. Also, I didn't want Kaylee home alone after Tony moves. Stephanie needed to get back to her home anyway for a few weeks before school starts. She was very happy about this news.

SATURDAY, AUGUST 21, 2010

Day 30, rehab 3

When I arrived home, I was really disappointed as to how work was not done at home. The garden was full of weeds, and grass was extremely long. I had no idea it would be this bad.

The girls were excited to show me the family pictures that Karen, our youth director had taken this past June. Kevin and I hadn't had an opportunity to view them yet due to the circumstances. Karen had dropped them off at our home for me to take down to Rochester to show Kevin on Sunday. Not only that, but she went through ALL of the pictures that she had taken and picked quite a few of the best ones out and printed them for us. She printed a couple of 8X10's and numerous 5X7's for us to display. She gave us the CD of all of the pictures for us to use as we chose. She picked

173

9 pictures out and put them in a collage frame that said "Family, It's the little moments that make life big." I realized at a later date, how long this must have taken her. When I needed to print a couple of pictures from the CD that she had given us, I couldn't believe how hard it was to do this. I mean, she had taken a couple hundred pictures in June. I was in awe at the wonderful job and gift that she had given to us. I was touched that someone would share their talent and so much time for us once again.

Today was the day that my firstborn was leaving home. Tony and I were able to ride up together and have some quality alone time on the three-and-a-half-hour car ride. Kaylee and Steph followed behind in my truck. We got to see his room and campus and have lunch together before heading back home. It was really nice that the girls were able to come with us.

Our friends Judy and Chris and their kids Ryan and Erin were at the campus already. They were done moving their son Ben in already. It was so nice for them to be there for us. They made sure they were available to help get some of the things in the dorm and support me by making sure that they were available in case I needed help handling all of the details that remained. Everything went smoothly.

When we came back home from taking Tony to college, I was able to enjoy some time on the tractor and the outdoors. I missed working outside and really needed this to relax and get my mind off Kevin.

SUNDAY, AUGUST 22, 2010

Day 31, rehab 4

I had a nice night in my own bed at home. I woke up refreshed, did chores, and visited with the girls before heading back down to Rochester. When I arrived in Kevin's room, his smile was radiant. He really missed me and was glad I was back. It's like at that very moment, we were both relieved to be together again. He is my soul mate, and I love him so much!

I pulled out the package of pictures that were given to us. I remember seeing how much Kevin was studying each and every one of them as he looked through the envelope of pictures. After he had completed this, I brought out the collage frame. He couldn't believe how beautiful this was and was so thankful for the wonderful gift.

We were able to find the perfect spot in his room to display this so we could see it at all times. Pictures are like a thousand words. The kids are far away from us and it was nice to see pictures of them throughout the day.

TUESDAY, AUGUST 24, 2010, 4:12 P.M.

Day 33, rehab 6

Today was another roller coaster day here at Rochester. Kevin feels pretty good and is doing quite well considering but is still very weak.

Kevin's platelets are doing well at 38. His white cells count is down to 0.5, and his hemoglobin is down to 7.9. This is not very good news at all. What's happening? Is he going backward again?

Kevin will be given red blood cells tonight via IV and two types of antibiotics and an antifungal medicine. So far, no tests have come back positive for anything on any cultures, but they don't want to take any chances at all.

The doctors had been concerned that throughout all of Kevin's struggles and this terrible disease, he might have injured his spine. Because of this, they gave Kevin an MRI this morning to see if they could find anything of concern. The results from the test showed no change from the January MRIs. This is good news for us. The bone marrow doctor did remark that they think that Kevin's stem cells are starting to graft in his system. Up and down, up and down. His cells are down, but the doctor thought that they were grafting? I'm confused.

I will keep in touch with you all as this progresses.

Starrla is a writer for our local newspaper back home. She had contacted me and wanted approval for her to do a story on our journey. I appreciated this and told her that I would work on getting her the facts.

Thanks for your additional prayers!

WEDNESDAY, AUGUST 25, 2010, 1:27 A.M.

Day 34, rehab 7, first e-mail

I went to the Ronald McDonald House today to get some information to pass on to Starrla for the newspaper article. I believe that there are people out there that don't know about houses like these. Possibly someone out there that could use a place like this when they or someone they know are in need. What better way to let others know than the newspaper.

When I stopped at the front desk of the Ronald McDonald house, the sweetest older gentleman greeted me with a smile. He asked me how I was, and I told him that I needed to find hope again. He told me to get down on my knees and pray. I told him that I have done this and still have nothing. I felt nothing at all.

Right now, at this very moment, as I'm typing this, I had the feeling in my head as a reminder, *O ye of so little faith!*

Kevin's fever has been ranging from 101 to 102.5. His blood pressure has been low, and he is boiling up and has chills. I feel like throwing up. I have a huge headache *again*! We can't sleep. It's dark in the room, and the doctors have a table outside Kevin's room door with a number of books. I don't know if they were research books or what they were. Are they reading up on how to best handle Kevin's situation? Many doctors are keeping a steady watch on Kevin. They are very concerned with his health. I think Kevin's scared.

Again, I feel like throwing up right now. Is it nerves? Am I sick? I am eating crackers and drinking Sierra Mist as I'm typing this letter. It's late right now, and I don't know who to call. I have many friends that have offered an ear to listen any time of day. I am hoping that the time difference in Nashville is earlier than Minnesota. I took the chance and called my cousin, Jolene, to talk to her. I think she would understand it if I was calling at a wrong time.

After our conversation, I went into the chapel and fell to my knees, crying and praying for Kevin. I am lost! I know God will carry Kevin, me, and the family through this. He's done a good job so far, and I can't lose hope or my faith. I need to take the time to sit, be still, rest my mind, pray, hope, and cry.

WEDNESDAY, AUGUST 25, 2010

Day 34, rehab 7/Methodist Hospital, second time
Day 1, second e-mail

Well, as far as Kevin goes, he must love it down here because he was transferred back to Methodist Hospital today. They did the transfer so the hematology and the bone marrow transplant doctors could keep a closer eye on him.

Kevin was told by his doctor that he is glad to see Kevin's positive attitude. He wished more patients were like that. This doctor had also read and commented on Kevin's board that's posted in his hospital room. This board included some facts about Kevin for the hospital staff to know a little more about him. The doctor then told us that when he read this board, he wasn't surprised with Kevin's attitude as soon as he read that Kevin is a Christian. Kevin agreed with this statement.

Kevin's temperature continues to go up. Now he had told us of a pain he gets when he lies in bed for a while. It's the same spot that he had pain in January when he had a blood clot in his lung.

Do you remember all of those times lately when I have said that I have no more hope? Well, lately, I have been feeling that Kevin keeps getting sick because of me. It is my fault. You see, I thought that because I was feeling like there's no hope, it was like I didn't have the faith that God would heal Kevin. I was searching for hope for a couple of weeks now, but it wasn't coming to me. I couldn't find it.

This morning, I was visiting with my mother on the phone. She told me four simple words that changed it all for me. These words were "Don't beat yourself up." After I hung up the phone, I realized that Jesus wouldn't want me to be hurt and blame myself for any of this. Instead, Jesus would want to put his arms around me and console me. These feelings I had were not true at all. I denounced them ASAP, and I won't feel like that again! Guess what?! The positive Karen is *back* and stronger than ever!

Then I read an e-mail that my friend, Kim, had sent me earlier that day. It was like déjà vu! She e-mailed me that she had been beating herself up, questioning her faith. Now, remember, I hadn't even e-mailed this letter yet. At the time I read her e-mail, I realized that I had never been alone in this struggle and maybe others didn't have a mother to tell them these simple words yet, so here they are! "Don't beat yourself up!"

Jesus wants to help you! Let's get back in the saddle and get things done! I will update you as soon as test results start coming up. Take care! I'm going to quit this letter and be still and pray on my knees because I know God is listening and I need help.

THURSDAY, AUGUST 26, 1:31 A.M.

Day 35, Methodist Hospital, second time, day 2

First of all, I would like to ask for prayers for my parents. My mom has been going through more than most would care due to her ankle replacements. She went in yesterday due to complications. Her previous surgery and treatment failed. They needed to do another surgery yesterday. My dad told me last night that five out of seven pins in her ankle had been broken for some time now and it wasn't discovered until yesterday. The surgery yesterday went from 8:00 a.m. to 3:00 p.m. The scans of this ankle that were taken in the past never showed any broken pins. She has endured a ton of pain this whole time.

My dad has a bad back but still has been getting my mom and grandmother around. Both of these fine women have been in wheelchairs for quite a while now. It's not just getting them and driving them somewhere. It's getting them into the car, folding, and lifting the wheelchairs and then repeating this all over again when you get to your destination. I am concerned that he is getting tired. Please pray for strength and healing for them all.

Today the medical staff planned on redoing some blood tests and a bone marrow biopsy on Kevin. They want to see if they can find something that's causing all of these problems.

I haven't been sleeping well at all. I am very tired. I feel like puking at times, and the days and nights seem to last forever! I feel like I'm in prison at times. I sure hope this doesn't take much longer! I have a seasonal job at Carlson's Apple Orchard. I have very understanding bosses and they are easy to work with. I was planning on working six days a week most weeks this year. This isn't too bad, considering that the restaurant is only open four months, August through Thanksgiving.

Rhonda's e-mail:

Hello!
I see that you are having some frustrations about Kevin heading back to the hospital because of his unknown temp.
Here is another scripture for you:

Being strengthened with all power according to His glorious might so that you may have great endurance and patience. Colossians 1:11

It is impossible for us to understand the true meaning of suffering unless we have endured it ourselves. Suffering is not something you can

177

learn from a book or a class. Suffering and the strength, endurance and patience that you will need to get through the trials in life can only be learned from Christ. After all, He is the one who suffered and died for us . . . He completely understands things that no one else can. When you feel weak turn to Christ and he will teach you how to be strong as this battle with Kevin continues.

Have a great day!

Rhonda

FRIDAY, AUGUST 27, DAY 36

Methodist Hospital, second time, day 3

The doctor's have not told us any new information yet. They have been giving Kevin the maximum amount of antibiotics that they can. They need to fight the infection that is killing all of his white cells. They also gave Kevin an injection of a drug that will increase production of the white cells that are currently living. This will hopefully keep enough white cells into his system while other cells are being killed with this infection. At the time, his white cell count jumped to 0.9. Kevin has a very upset stomach and is getting steroids for this.

I know there is more. I just can't think anymore. Each day blends together here, as I'm sure most of you know.

SATURDAY, AUGUST 28, DAY 37

Methodist Hospital, second time, day 4

Kevin had fevers and shakes pretty bad the last few days and nights. This had really been concerning me.

Today seemed to make a turn toward the better once again. Kevin's stem cell count jumped to 4.1 today. This is unbelievably wonderful news. The doctors are really pleased with the success. We were told that we might be able to move Kevin back to the transplant house as soon as tomorrow. This really surprised both of us. We just got back to the hospital four days ago.

Our friends Chris and Judy stopped in to see Kevin today. Judy is a nurse. She told me that she doesn't specialize in this kind of illness but would be more than happy to be a standby nurse on call for us when we get home if we need. This really made me feel better. I believe that we probably will be fine but is really nice to know that we have someone to lean on if we need.

Kevin has been in the amends before, and as you know, things have been known to change quickly.

Al and Dede brought our girls down here with them again for a visit.

SUNDAY, AUGUST 29, 2010, 8:38 A.M.

Day 38, Methodist Hospital, second time, day 5
Transplant house 1

He finally had a good night last night.

Kevin's white cell count jumped to 12.3! I guess the drug to increase cell production really worked! Praise God! Believe this or not. They are going to release us back to the transplant house today! What a shock! The doctors feel that Kevin will heal better there. He will be monitored daily for the coming days ahead to see if he stays in stable condition. If he stays in good health, we might be able to come home in a few days. It's unbelievable. How can they think that he will be fine to leave in a few days? Hasn't he proved a number of times that he keeps getting sick? Don't they want to give it a week or two yet? What am I supposed to do when he gets sick and we're at home?

Kevin and I really didn't talk much after the news of our move. Both of our minds were going a million miles a minute. We were a little nervous and not sure how we felt. One would think that both of us would be jumping up and down for joy, but we're not. We are scared. I'm used to the nurses coming every two hours, one hour, or even half hour to check on Kevin's vitals. They make sure that he is okay. I'm not in charge. All of a sudden, I'm on my own with no check between visits. It's *not* very comforting at all.

My sister, Penny, Alan and their sons, Jeff and Brent, came down to visit. This made the day go much smoother for us. They were excited and surprised to hear of the news that Kevin was getting out of the hospital. They made sure that they waited for us to be dismissed so they could help me get everything back to the transplant house.

You know, the medical staff may tell you that you're getting released from the hospital in the morning, but then it took up to five hours for the actual release. There was a lot of paperwork I guess that needed to get done prior to our release, and they didn't know it would take this long. You want to get out not because you think you should but knowing that you need to go because the doctors released you. You are trying to make a plan of action when you move, but just wait, wait, and wait some more.

After we got settled at the transplant house, I called my boss and told them that I would be coming home soon and would ready for work. I realize that it was getting awfully close to my start date but wasn't prepared for the news I received. Unfortunately I was informed that I would not be hired for full time this year. I was crushed by this news. I cried and cried and cried. I needed that job. I needed to make some money to help with the medical bills. I needed to have a purpose.

The bosses felt that due to Kevin's ups and downs with his health, it would be a good business decision to hire someone else to fill my position at this time. If anything were to go wrong again with Kevin after we were home, I would not be able to work and they would be short a waitress. They did, however, tell me that they would hire me to fill in for those who needed certain days off. I really do understand and agree with their decision. I know that they felt bad, and I realized that this really was necessary. I mean at this point, who knows when we will be coming home anyway.

I'll e-mail you with any news we hear today or tomorrow as to our release date. Thanks for your prayers.

Monday, August 30, 2010

Day 39, transplant house, second time, day 2

Kevin was really quiet again today. I'm sure a lot of stuff is going through his mind just like it is mine. Sometimes, I wonder if he doesn't feel good, would he tell me.

The two weeks prior to our release from the Mayo were concerning Penny, Vicki, and me due to my extreme dizziness. I became so off balance and couldn't control my shakes and tremors when I walked too fast. I don't want to worry Kevin, so I'm trying to get over this on my own. Is it the addition and reduction of my old and new medications? Is it stress or is it just the elevators and my injured inner ear again?

Tuesday, August 31, 2010

Day 40, transplant house, second time, day 3

Kevin's white cell count has decreased again. Kevin's cell count was now back down to 7.1. I was alarmed at first but then was reminded that the normal cell count amount is 3.5 to 10. He is right where he needs to be. The doctors were not concerned at all about this. Actually, they expected this to happen. Remember this past Friday when they gave Kevin an IV of growth factor? This was for the cells to multiply. They multiplied enough cells to carry a reserve amount for such a reduction. This way, if the infection would keep killing the cells, there would be some in his system already to replace them.

Wednesday, September 1, 2010, 7:09 a.m.

Day 41, transplant house, second time, day 4

Sunday night through Tuesday night went well for Kevin, keeping a low-grade temperature. His platelet count also remained at a consistent level during this time.

Things are getting tense between Kevin and me right now. I think we are scared to be set free from this place. We are not being patient with each other at all. I'm trying to plan on how to pack the rest of our stuff up for the trip back home. We still are unaware if we will get to come home this week or not. How do we plan when we don't know?

My sister, Vicki, came to visit today and was a ton of help to me. She helped me pack up stuff from the transplant house that I knew I wouldn't need during the rest of our stay here and organized it all in the Suburban for our trip home. She is a great packer and saved me a lot of time and frustration.

I purchased a walker for Kevin and, after some time, found the correct place to rent a wheelchair so our insurance would cover the cost. I wanted to get this all done now so when we're home, we are set for anything.

I, of course, was up way too early again today. I was having bad dreams again and yelling at people in my sleep. I was sick of waking myself up, so I just got up and did laundry, etc.

Today was a really big day for us, with appointments starting at 10:45 a.m. and going through 4:00 p.m. These appointments educated us on what is necessary to continue treatment at home, cleanliness needs, and future appointments. Kevin also had a final cell-count numbers check.

When we came back to the Gift Transplant House today, I felt like my eyes were going wacky. I was so light-headed and started to feel like I was losing my balance from time to time. I think it's the new medication, plus riding so many elevators today could have disrupted my inner ear again.

I called my specialist in the cities and told him that I couldn't waitress in this condition! I understood him to tell me to *quit all* of my medications for two weeks to clean my system out. Then we'd start all over at that time! The medicines I needed to quit included medications for arthritis, nerves, and headaches, which included a type of antidepressant that I have been on for about seven years. This should be fun! I had no choice. There is no way I could even drive the car home in this condition. Oh, well, life goes on with daily challenges. My only goal right now is to help my husband get on the road to recovery.

There have been many patients at this transplant house who have come back from their final appointments with the bad news of needing to stay another couple of days. We're hoping that will *not* be our case. If all goes well, we are planning on leaving tomorrow, midmorning, and coming home. It will be so nice for both of us to be in familiar surroundings with our kids and animals once again.

This is a recap of our year so far: Between Abbott Hospital and the Mayo Clinic, Kevin has been away from home for eighty-seven days this year. He has been in the hospital for twenty-two days, in the ICU for thirty days, in rehab for seven days, and in the transplant house for twenty-eight days. Funny how at times it seems like it was longer than this.

Being at the Mayo Clinic was a very humbling experience for me! Everyone who thinks that they have it so bad should go for a visit to a local hospital, nursing home, or the Mayo Clinic even once. Keep your eyes open to seeing those who are less fortunate than you and give thanks for life.

We are so appreciative for all of the support that we have been shown throughout this journey. God has surely blessed us and has given Kevin a second chance at life. I pray that you also have come out of this journey of ours with something positive to impact your life.

As you probably know, Kevin will probably need a lot of rest for a while once we are at home. We will hopefully see you all soon. Definitely at volleyball or football games.

I'll e-mail with updates as Kevin's healing process continues.

Praise God for all things, and remember to live every day like it was your last.

We want to thank you all again for all of your prayers.

Chapter 11

THE NEW BEGINNING AND STRUGGLES

Day 42, transplant house, second time
Day 5, Kevin home 1

Kevin had his last blood draw this morning, and the results were good. What a miracle! What a blessing! Why aren't we jumping up and down and so excited that we can't quit smiling? Instead, we're both really focused on getting home. Our minds are racing.

I am stressed with finishing packing, cleaning our food storage area, refrigerator shelf, and freezer tote at the transplant house. I need to make sure that I have followed all of the checkout instructions of cleanliness. We have a check out deadline time that I need to meet too. I also was trying to get the truck loaded as quickly as possible. I didn't want to take too much time at the parking spot in the front of the Gift of Life Transplant House. The shuttle bus comes through there periodically to pick up patients and caregivers, and I didn't want to be in the way.

There was a young lady who was a caretaker staying at the Gift House and saw that I was having a difficult time pulling the huge cart filled with our belongings. She was kind and helped me get everything to the truck. That's one of the nice things about this place. Everyone understands and is going through similar stresses and concerns.

Once we got on the road for home, it was smooth sailing. Traffic was light, and so was the conversation as far as the amount of it. We were home by one thirty. As soon as we arrived, the dogs came barreling out of the house. They were so happy to see us and barked and wiggled so much for quite some time. I helped Kevin into the house, and the kids were waiting for us with the biggest smiles. It was so nice to see everyone together again.

I couldn't believe it when I came into the house. Everything was *immaculate*! Clean! It even smelled nice! I am so thankful to Lisa for cleaning and disinfecting our

ENTIRE home and to Judy who cleaned our carpets. This was no small task! As we walked into the living room, on the fireplace mantle was a wonderful poster that the kids made, welcoming Kevin home.

As soon as Kevin was able to get comfortable on the couch, and we greeted one another, I wanted to get unpacked. Everyone else wanted to rest and visit. It was like I needed my journey home to be completed, and nobody else understood that. I had food in the truck that needed to get out and put away. It seemed as though nobody was happy to see me. Nobody missed me and nobody hugged me either. I was very hurt. No, hurt doesn't even come close. I was crushed. Then I come in with all of our boxes and junk from living down at Rochester for the summer. I felt extremely frustrated because now I messed up this immaculate cleaning job already. Now I'd need to reorganize this stuff into our home.

My friend that I met at the transplant house told me not to come home expecting to do it all again, like I did before our trip to Rochester. She told me it takes time to heal. I only thought Kevin needed to heal. I had no idea that I would also need some time to heal and get back into the swing of things. Do you think I'd listen?! As soon as I got home, I was concerned how I'd keep the house this clean, how I was going to go to work at the Orchard, do all of the yard, and harvest the garden.

Later on in the day, I had a strong desire to leave. I felt trapped. Like I couldn't breathe or focus on what to do with myself. I didn't realize that this hurt Kevin's feelings. Can you imagine your wife needing to get away from you and the house? I felt like nobody understood me, nobody loved me, and I just couldn't please anyone. I went to a friend's house for a couple of hours figuring that when I came back home, things would feel better for me. I was wrong.

I felt bad feeling selfish and sensitive. Why doesn't Kevin and/or any of the kids even think of all that I had endured this past summer too? It's almost like all of a sudden, I'm not satisfied with my life and all that I have been given. I truly am thankful. It's just that I don't act like it right now.

I tried to ignore this as best as I could. The kids have been through a ton this past summer too, and I really need to give them some slack, but I am struggling with this too.

FRIDAY, SEPTEMBER 3

Kevin home 2

Kevin felt pretty good yesterday but took a turn for the worse today around noon or so. His stomach became upset, his appetite was totally gone, he had quite a bit of diarrhea, and he threw up and had a low-grade temperature. He became *very* chilled and miserable. I had him covered up with two thick tie blankets because he kept asking to be warmer. I added a rag rug and some towels to keep the blankets free of vomit. His body was shaking and trembling terribly! This continued throughout the day and evening. Put it this way. Friday was a *long* night again with no or little sleep. I was scared. I periodically checked his temperature, making sure that it didn't go overly high again like it did in August.

SATURDAY, SEPTEMBER 4

Kevin home 3

I called the Mayo hospital on Saturday morning explaining all that had transpired. I was instructed to bring Kevin to Rochester immediately. When I told them how far away we were, they told me to take him to the Buffalo emergency department as soon as possible. We needed to make sure his numbers and vitals were okay. Kevin was reluctant to go because he said that he wasn't feeling quite as bad as he did yesterday. He felt this trip to the hospital would be a waste of time. Being as the Mayo Clinic told us to go, and it was a holiday weekend, I decided that this was a necessary trip. We really didn't know if he was having another setback, and I didn't want to take any chances.

The blood tests at the emergency room came back wonderfully! We were so pleased, relieved, and thankful. The results were even better than at our release appointment from the Mayo Clinic. Amazing! The doctors don't have an answer as to why Kevin felt like this. They said that it is possible that his body was retaliating to all of the drugs that needed to be given to him during his illness. It could also be attributed to the stress he has been in.

As soon as we got home from the emergency room, all I wanted to do was get out of the house again. I couldn't think. I was anxious, needing to be alone, upset, and depressed. I was miserable. Was I feeling like this because I was afraid? Was I feeling like this because I finally have someone else who can take over for me as caretaker and give me some freedom? What is going on?

I told Kaylee that I needed her to give me a break from caretaking and stay with Kevin while I was gone. I think she was surprised at my request. I had to try anything to get my head straight. I asked Stephanie to come with me grocery shopping and out to lunch with a couple of friends. This was really a nice and relaxing outing for me, and I was glad to have one on one with Stephanie for some time. When I returned home, I still felt the need to get out again! I don't understand. It's like I was trying to run away from something. I plainly didn't want to be home at all!

I will pull myself together, but I need you to please pray with me that this passes soon. I keep telling myself that this is all part of life.

SUNDAY, SEPTEMBER 5

Kevin home 4

Kevin's appetite seems to be good today, and he seems to be feeling much better. I am so thankful for the wonderful friends and family that have been listening to my emotions as I am trying to cope with all of the changes, ups and downs, and stresses. I have become depressed. I have been crying a lot, have been very disappointed in the upkeep of the farm, have been emotional, and to top it off, have had continuous headaches.

I am quiet because I'm afraid of what I will say now. I didn't know what I wanted or why I was crying. I also was in the full swing of menopause, which seemed to be really fun like a lot of you already know. I would never have thought that there would be new stresses when returning home from Rochester. I remember some stress from returning home from Abbott, but I was closer to home during that time and could make short visits home. I think these factors made it easier for all of us then. Also the Abbott NW stay was only twenty-nine days away versus fifty-eight days in Rochester.

Think of those who come back from war, from having a stroke, from being transferred away from home for some time due to work, a separation of marriage, and coming back home to try again. The stresses of getting responsibilities and priorities back to the way they were before they left are tough. The emotions and the trust might be issues also. These feelings that I have been experiencing are not only subjected to the weak. They also aren't prejudice to religion or race. People throughout the whole universe experience this. Many people try to ignore it, cover it up, don't understand it, or hold it in. It's just possible that this might hit too close to home for some of you.

I know through all of the miracles that I have already experienced that even when things seem to get worse, we still need to thank God for the positive things that happen. I am thankful that Kevin got home safely and is probably in remission from this cancer. I am thankful that I am able to stay home and care for him. I am thankful that our house is still standing when we got home. I am thankful that the kids and the animals are healthy. Deep down, I am thankful that we are together as a family again. The farm work will always be there tomorrow or the next day. I am thankful that I have the property to even have farmwork on and am healthy enough to do the work myself.

Karen update

If I want to reach out to people and be an advocate for others in their struggles, I need to be open and share mine!

It's late. I can't sleep. I'm crying again! I feel alone, empty, miserable, disappointed, sad, helpless, unloved, uncontrollable, and selfish and all in pieces and don't know how to pick myself up and put myself together again. I've been trying so hard to stay strong for myself, Kevin, the kids, and my family so they don't worry about me since December 2009. I succeeded only because of your prayers and God had carried me the whole way. Together strong!

Right now, at this moment, I feel like God just abandoned me. It's possible that I've been asking God to help me and I have been too tied up in asking and talking about it and not listening to what he wanted me to know. I tried to overlook this feeling and ignore it, but it just sits in my head and I keep thinking of it over and over again.

Last Thursday, I was already told by a family member that I'm annoying. I guess I asked too many questions the minute I got home. I admit that I wanted help unpacking and was probably a little bit bossy. I missed the kids and now was back home and wanted to be back in charge and take care of them. Maybe I was too overbearing. This was such a change back for everyone. Kevin was getting upset and irritated. He had told me, "Sorry for getting sick" (because I'm depressed) and "Just take the pills you were told to quit so you stop being like this."

It seems like nobody even thinks of asking what's wrong or how can they help me feel better? How about a hug or just holding me in their arms and telling me that we will get through this together? Is everyone afraid of me? Is everyone confused and ignore me because they don't know what to do? Why don't I ask for a hug? Why can't I tell them what's wrong? Do I even know other than I'm depressed? Do I know what I need or want? I feel so alone and abandoned.

Stephanie took the keys from the vehicles because she didn't believe me that I promised not to leave at 12:30 a.m. on Sunday night. She was afraid of where I was going to go and what I was going to do. She thought I was going to commit suicide. That poor girl! What did I put her through? Right now, I really don't care if I'm alive or not. Don't worry, I want to end my life, but I'm not strong enough to commit suicide. Just think if I could do it. I wouldn't have any more pain, frustration, or sadness. I just don't care about anything anymore. Nothing feels good to me at all! I know that this too shall pass, but it sure seems like it's taking a long time. Talk about time standing still! It just never goes or leaves me alone! The days and nights keep going on and on and on and on. My heart is broken.

TUESDAY, SEPTEMBER 7

Today was Kevin's first appointment for blood draw. The results will get faxed to the Mayo Clinic for evaluation. We don't know what the numbers of his white cell count is yet, but we aren't concerned at all. Kevin was given testing and instructions on his blood-thinner dose changes and needs to go back again on Friday for a checkup.

Tonight was our first volleyball game for the season, and it was so wonderful to see and talk to friends that we have greatly missed. You know, I thought this outing would help me get out of this slump I'm in, but it was just easier to ignore it for a short while. It came back again as soon as I got home.

Kevin is still really weak, and I know that Kevin is looking forward to the day that he can walk up steps and sit in the bleachers to be in the middle of everyone he wants to talk to. He loves giving crap to others and, of course, gives his game comments.

When we left Rochester, Kevin was instructed that he needed to wear his mask everywhere other than at our house. We were notified today during his doctors' appointment that due to the good numbers, Kevin doesn't have to wear his face mask anymore, other than at the clinic or hospital. He still shouldn't be around people that have any kind of illness or large groups. If he needs to be, he will need his mask. I still am concerned and cautious about this, yet because we haven't been home that long. I understand how uncomfortable the mask is and also understand why he doesn't like wearing it, but it is still a protector.

Thank you for all of your prayers, thoughts, concerns, and well wishes because without them, this would have been a much more difficult journey.

WEDNESDAY, SEPTEMBER 8

Kevin is very weak today but determined to get back in the groove ASAP. He is a good patient and follows rules pretty well so far. He is happy to be home, but his mind is moving a million miles per hour thinking about too much stuff. He wants to get back to work soon.

As of now, the doctors say that the cancer, not Kevin's cancer—we don't take ownership of this, is in remission. We will continue to be monitored and treated as needed by going to the Buffalo clinic to get occasional blood draws and stabilize his blood thinner.

We will need to go back to Rochester on Kevin's hundredth-day post transplant for a checkup. This will be in about two months from now.

THURSDAY, SEPTEMBER 9, 2010, 11:18 P.M.

Karen chapter 2

Quite often this summer the kids told me how much they missed Kevin. Whenever I asked for them to stay overnight with me in Rochester, they didn't want to. They wanted to go home. I was confused. Why wouldn't they want to stay down here and have extra time with him? They already made the drive.

At times, when I'd call them, I would hear how irritating I am to the kids when I asked if things were done at home. I was talked to like I was bothering them or keeping them from something more important.

I was trying to keep both places under control. I wanted to feel like I was still a part of their lives, even though I was so far away from them. I understand that they felt like they were in control of things, but I wasn't there to see it. Was I controlling? Were they disrespectful? I was angry about this at times. I need to admit that Kevin or I didn't realize the difficulty the kids faced emotionally with this cancer diagnosis until this past August.

We had told our coordinator at the Mayo Clinic about the struggles that we have had with the kids this past year. She presented us with information that really opened our eyes.

I didn't feel that the added pressures and responsibilities that were put on the kids were too much for them to deal with, but the duration might have played a huge part in this. This is the second time in one year that they have been faced with the unknown and no parent there to support and comfort them. They were totally on their own.

I wish I would have been prepared for this. Maybe a person just can't be prepared, but I'm hoping that my letter just might prepare at least one other person.

I know I am blessed, I know God is watching me, I know God is using my honest expression to reach out to others, I know I am loved, and I know I will be all right!

At times, I feel like a hypocrite, writing like this after all of those e-mails this past summer. Each one I wrote was true and from the heart. It's just I'm only human and am at a weak stage right now and need your prayers. The ups and downs are unreal. One day I'm fine, and the next is totally different. What a rollercoaster ride this is.

I haven't kept up on taking care of myself since December 2009. I have been caring for everyone else but me. I can't be dizzy anymore, so I decided to tell the doctor that I started back on my inner ear medication today because it's necessary. This should help a ton with my dizziness. I also decided to try to get back into exercising. I realize that this will be a great help with my depression and 20 pound weight gain.

TUESDAY, SEPTEMBER 14, 2010, 12:42 P.M.

Kevin home 2

Kevin has been feeling kind of sick in the afternoons lately with an upset stomach. We are pretty sure it might be from the pills he has to take.

Kevin got into the truck by himself today with no help at all. A few days ago, he had been walking a little bit with no cane or walker. He is very weak, but he makes it. I am very proud of his determination. I asked him to write out a couple of bills today to help me out. He filled out two envelopes with return addresses and had enough already. I didn't think his hands and fingers would still be this weak!

This week, Thursday, Kevin will start a new medicine called Bactrim. This will change his blood thickness and was given to prevent him from getting pneumonia. He only needs to take this pill for about two months. If we would choose not to take this pill, we would need to go to the Mayo Clinic to get a treatment on a nebulizer for one and a half hours each month.

Kevin's appetite has been really good. I enjoy seeing him eat and not be picky about what it is. We don't need to go to the doctor now until next week, and we will just keep plugging away and take care of each other.

Kevin update

FRIDAY, SEPTEMBER 17, 2010, 10:01 A.M.

Do you believe that we've been home for two weeks? Well, other than one emergency visit, Kevin's health and strength have been getting better each day. He has been standing and walking without a walker and cane more and more, pushing himself to get stronger. I haven't needed to give him a goose to get into the truck for a number of days now. His appetite is good, and he has been sleeping well at night for all I know. I have not needed to give him a shower anymore. He has been strong enough to stand alone without support and is just getting better as each day passes.

Another gentleman that we met down in Rochester is only a few weeks ahead of Kevin and commented to us that he too is struggling with getting stronger. It's a very slow process, but we need to be patient. It is nice to hear from someone else to compare our strengths and weaknesses.

Kevin and Karen update

WEDNESDAY, OCTOBER 6, 2010, 10:35 P.M.

Kevin started going in to work for a couple of hours a day to start. I think this will be very healing for him to get back into his normal life. You can only sit and watch TV for so long. A person can go stir crazy. Kevin was given the okay to quit his magnesium and potassium now because his electrolytes are at a good stage and his cells are no longer eating up these nutrients. He is tired a lot and has a sore neck quite often. It isn't helping that he is not sitting in the wheelchair with his neck support at the games anymore. He has sore hips at times but, at the same time, is feeling good to be in remission.

We are so blessed with friends and family that are still helping us with so many different things. Friendship is a blessing for us to receive and give.

Thanks for your prayers and I will update again in the future.

THURSDAY, OCTOBER 14, 2010, 10:53 A.M.

Kevin has started going in to work now from 10:00 a.m. to 5:00 p.m. each day. This is more than the doctor wants him to do, but he seems fine.

It's been a long time that we have been dealing with health issues in this house. Sometimes, when issues go on and on and on and on, which is how I feel this issue was, most of the time, people forget about the problem their friend had and just go on with their lives. Do you know that we are still getting cards and special words of encouragement? We are very touched by the love that still surrounds us.

With no surprise, the community is once again stepped up and helped us. They hosted a hot dish supper with salads, desserts, and beverages from 4:00 to 7:00 p.m. Friday, October 22, at the Lions Hall in Howard Lake. There was a freewill offering for the meal. The proceeds benefited us. Wow!

There was one bill that we received from the hospital. I remember looking at it from time to time and wondering when and how I was going to pay for it. Amazingly, the amount of money earned from the Lions benefit that they had for us was almost *exactly* the same amount we owed on this bill. What a blessing and a gift!

God has blessed us with many riches of family, friends, and even those who just know us by name. He has blessed us with *you*! Thank you for being there and letting God work through you.

TUESDAY, NOVEMBER 9, 2010

Day 100 for Kevin

Thank you, God! It's already been a hundred days since Kevin's transplant. Life is different now, and like Kevin said this morning, it will be until the day we pass away. This is nothing we can't handle because we know God wouldn't allow this if we couldn't.

Did Kevin's desire to push himself lessen because of the duration of the struggle? Is he doing too much at work, leaving no energy for himself to heal? I want to help, but don't know what more I can do. Watching Kevin each day walking weakly, having no energy to do anything, and no desire or ability, or so it seems, to improve his strength bothers me.

I read a few pages in the book *Finding Your Way Families and the Cancer Experience: A Guidebook.* It said in there that caretakers shouldn't feel guilty wanting to be at work instead of at home or just needing to get away or even to just be alone at times. I was relieved to read this. I'm so excited, nervous, and anxious to work at the Apple Orchard again this year, even if it's not full time. This will be my time to be out of the house and be able to make some much-needed money besides. I won't feel bad wanting to leave the house, Kevin, or the household responsibilities anymore.

To top it off, when we were down in Rochester this summer, there was a hailstorm at home that caused damage. I noticed all of the roofs being repaired in the area and called on a roofer to check our roofs. We found out that our house and the three outbuildings we have, needed complete roof replacement. The chimney cap on our house came off from the wind during the late-summer storm too. Whenever it rained after that, the water came down the fireplace and into Tony's bedroom in the basement. The carpet had been wet for sometime but nobody could figure out where the water was coming from including me. Fortunately when the roofers came over, I thought to show them this problem. We are very lucky that nobody got sick from the mold that had already grown. It took some arranging and phone calls, but everything from the insurance company to the repair details for this got figured out.

Last night, we arrived in Rochester for Kevin's appointment today at the Mayo Clinic. Kevin has given blood this morning, and after that, he was scheduled for a bone marrow biopsy. I forgot how much Kevin needed me with him. I was in the waiting room, and the nurse came out and said that Kevin asked her to get me. Isn't that nice? I felt needed at that time. The next step was the bone survey. This is x-rays of this skeletal system.

191

At three fifteen, we saw the doctor for the results of the day. Here it goes. The Myeloma cancer seems to still be in remission. They are still waiting on the bone biopsy report, which should be read in the next few days. The rest of the numbers from the tests are good. Thank you, God!

The average time frame for the Myeloma cancer to come back is two to three years. There is a study saying that by continuing the Revlimid medicine, the cancer remission could possibly keep for a long period of time, but that isn't proven. Kevin's doctor didn't feel it necessary for Kevin to do this because there are unnecessary side effects that could go along with this. He'd need to take extra pills, and his blood thinner would need to continue. When and if the cancer returns is the time that Kevin will go on medication.

Kevin's uric acid was high, and the doctors will recheck this in one week just in case it was misread. If it's still high, they will medicate at that time. Kevin's blood sugar is also a little high, so we need to keep track of this.

Kevin was given a bone marrow infusion today also. He has received this infusion already in the past to strengthen his bone marrow and will need to do it every three months. It is given intravenously for one and a half hours.

The doctor did write orders up for Kevin to do physical therapy for his neck pain and to get the proper exercises to strengthen him and give him more energy. This will also keep his aches and pains away more. The doctor did say walking twenty minutes or riding a bike each day will also help him heal.

THURSDAY, DECEMBER 2, 5:29 P.M.

Kevin has been sick for five days now. He feels like shit because his neck hurts. He doesn't want to go to the therapist for help because last year, when he went for his neck pain that we didn't know was a tumor, they could have *really* hurt him. He doesn't want to do therapy because he's tired, sore, and doesn't trust therapists anymore.

I look at him and he seems so sad, frustrated, and helpless at times. Then I think about this: *What if I had cancer? Even if it is in remission, it could be back tomorrow.* I know, Kevin says, he doesn't think about that, but is this true? Would I? Would you? Do the kids?

DECEMBER 20

I have written about my struggle with depression and suicidal thoughts in the past. I could have gone on and on writing about this, but it would have just been repetitive. Each story would have been different but, at the same token, repetitive. I have decided that instead of being repetitive, I would sum it all up in the following paragraphs.

I had many thoughts of how I could end my life. Jumping out of my moving vehicle was thought of the most. I remember calling a relative and telling them that I wanted to open the door and jump out of my truck as I was driving home one afternoon. This person didn't know what to say. Instead of talking me through this feeling, they totally changed the topic of our conversation. The next day I called them and said, "Do you realize that you ignored my call for help?" They felt really bad but told me, "I just didn't know what to say. I thought if I'd change the subject, you would get your mind off of what you wanted to do." I told them that I understood their reaction, but we can't be afraid to deal with this.

Nobody wants to talk about the subject of suicide. We are all afraid of it. Usually, we don't know how to approach this or know what to say unless you have gone through this yourself. There may be times that someone talks about how depressed they are over and over. Some may wonder if they are truly depressed or just sad because of how their life is going and are looking for attention. Then there are those who talk about their depression in hopes to get some help. Who do we decide to take seriously? Do we want to take that kind of chance?

DECEMBER 22

I hit rock bottom tonight. I have been having dealing suicidal thoughts from September through December. I have been unbearable to live with most of this time. If I would have remembered about the suicide help line, would I have called them? It is possible that I would not have because they are far away from me and it's not personable. I wouldn't be able to feel genuine love or care over the phone either. I probably would have had too much pride and felt I could handle this on my own. Was I too consumed in my life that I didn't ask or allow God to help me? I don't remember.

I was waiting for this night to come, but nobody could have ever prepared me for how bad it would be.

Kevin and I were on the way home from Christmas shopping tonight, and I felt an extremely strong desire to open the truck door and jump out again. It seemed to be a stronger presence of no self-worth than it had been in the past. I felt that I was making life miserable for Kevin and the kids. I can't do or say anything right anymore. I'm so depressed that I feel like vomiting quite often. To top this all off, I have struggled daily with even the littlest of tasks for many years now due to my head trauma and I'm really tired. I feel wore out. I don't want to deal with this pain and trial any longer. Everyone would be better off without me. Just end it now and I will be free from it all.

All of a sudden, I thought of the kids. I visualized them crying by my grave and realized that I wouldn't want to put them through this pain and sadness. They really do need me even if they don't know it now. What's happening here? How did it get this far? The Devil is trying to kill my relationship with my family and kill me along with that. I *won't* allow him to do this to me. I have to get my life back. How do I do this? I need help!

I prayed and instantly got renewed strength from God. I decided to work along with him to fix this mess. I denounced the Devil at that very moment and said to myself, *No! This would be the easy way out for me. This isn't the answer.*

Jeremiah 29:11: "For I know the plans I have for you, declares the Lord."
Never give the Devil a ride. He will want to take over the driving.

When we got home, I couldn't stop crying. We had to do something NOW! The kids were home, and Kevin realized that we needed to have a family meeting with all of us. I said, "I dug my hole so deep with you guys, and now how do I get myself out? How do I get you to love me again?" Kevin looked at me and said, "Karen, we love you very much. We'll get through this together."

After a couple days of pulling myself together and feeling regret and guilt with all that had occurred, I continued to try to start fresh. I decided to pull out the book I found when we were at the St. Mary's Rehab facility in Rochester. I had to start somewhere. This book was called *Understanding Brain Injury: A Guide for the Family*. I was hoping to learn something that I could do to help myself.

When I started reading this, I was in total awe. There were so many side effects emotionally and physically that I have been dealing with. I had always thought that it was just the way I was. Where was this book eight years ago? Why didn't I read this in August when we were at the rehab center? I couldn't believe it. So many of the things I struggle with are listed as possible side effects from my brain injury. This book isn't a "feel sorry for me that I have this problem" book. It is a book to teach me how to deal with these side effects. I felt that I would be able to cope with my current difficulties better if other daily struggles I experience were diminished.

I had been on medication for my extreme headaches for 8 years already. I didn't know that it included an anti-depressant. I had done a switch on medication mid August and had quit cold turkey on all of them for a couple weeks at the end of August beginning of September. Did this attribute to my problems?

I decided to share what I had learned from this book with Kevin and the kids. They were surprised too. They would say, "Hey, you do that all of the time." After I told them the side effect I told them what I needed to do in order to avoid this type of reaction. *Side effect example; Limited ability to focus, Has a hard time keeping up when topics change. What to do; ask the person to make the topic brief but VERY detailed; ask the person to look at you when speaking and reduce distractions.* We made a plan to work together.

Chapter 12

FINDING FAITH

Thursday, January 6, 2011

Kevin and I watched a minister on TV on Sunday that really rocked my thinking. I told God that I *really* needed his help and I know that I can't survive without him. This minister spoke and said, "If you feel sorry for yourself, *nobody cares*! Who doesn't have problems? How are others going to help you if you can't make yourself happy? You can't blame others for your depression. Are you depressed because of what somebody said to you? Does this make it their fault that you're depressed? You made yourself react like that. Get over it! Get happy. If you can't figure out a plan of action and take care of it, only you and God can get yourself out of depression."

Some depression is chemical, and medication is helpful in treating this, but you still would need the help of God and yourself to heal.

I realized that if my family hasn't been reacting to my needs, maybe they don't know what they are? How would they know unless I communicate these to them in detail? How am I going to be angry with them for not making me happy, when I don't make myself happy?

At that moment, I became determined to communicate better to my family and knew I needed a plan and a change. I felt like a huge burden lifted off of my shoulders instantly. I understood and knew that it was up to me to let God help me.

Sometimes, it's easier to keep issues to ourselves, and get upset because the men and/or women in our lives don't react like we want them to. It's like, then, we can have someone else to blame our bad feelings on and push it all on someone else instead of taking ownership to the issues at hand. I may be struggling right now because of a number of things. I will make it once again to the top with joy, happiness, and a stronger faith in my Lord Jesus Christ. We all need to work together, help each other, and love unconditionally.

Recently I started having attacks of breathing difficulties. This was really scary for me. I remember lying in bed one night, counting my breaths. I was confused as to why this was happening to me all of a sudden. I questioned whether I was going to die or not at times. I asked Kevin to take me to the emergency room, but he convinced me that they wouldn't be able to help me anyway. Not only this, but my headaches were terrible also. I was miserable and scared.

The next morning, the first thing I did was called my specialist. I told him what had been going on. He told me to see my family doctor as soon as possible and schedule an appointment to see a psychologist for medication of depression and anxiety. It's possible that the medication that I quit taking had helped me previously with anxiety also. He was hoping that the psychologist could also find something else to remedy my headaches.

FRIDAY, JANUARY 7, 2011

I went to see my family physician today. He did a number of tests on me and determined that he felt that I was experiencing anxiety attacks. This could be due to a lack of medications or stress. He wanted further testing done at the psychiatrist office at my appointment. I was prescribed a medication to help relieve this and was instructed on how to deal with breathing difficulties until the medicine became effective.

KAREN'S SECOND JOURNAL IN 2011

TUESDAY, JANUARY 11, 2011

I went to church for prayer ministry today. I felt this was the best place to go in order for me to get a fresh look and plan of action for help. Not only did I need help for myself, but also my whole family needed help.

Kevin has been really quiet lately. It's like he's just sitting there waiting to die or get the cancer back. I feel that he doesn't feel that he's man of the house anymore because I have taken over so many of his responsibilities due to his limitations. He is possibly strong enough to take some of them over but could be scared at the same time as to if he can do the job as well as he would like to.

What I got out of this time at church was that maybe Kevin was depressed too. I talked to him about that at night, and he said, "No, I'm not depressed." He got mad at me because he said that I always psychoanalyze everything. After some time had passed that same night and he had time to think, out of nowhere, he said, "Maybe I am a little depressed and I don't even know it." This made so much sense to both of us.

We also discussed that I didn't feel that Kevin was pushing himself to get stronger at all anymore. He agreed with this statement and told me that he would pay attention to this more each day. We agreed that he would start to try to take over some of the man of the house's responsibilities. This will not only help me out quite a bit, but I think this will make him feel better about himself also.

Before I went to bed last night, I read this card I have that has a prayer on it. It really hit me when I read the part about praying for myself. This is what it says:

> Make me my husband's helpmate, companion, champion, friend, and support. Help me to create a peaceful, restful, safe place for him to come home to. Teach me how to take care of myself and stay attractive to him. Grow me into a creative and confident woman who is rich in mind, soul, and spirit. Make me the kind of woman he can be proud to say is his wife. I lay all of my expectations at your cross, Lord Jesus. I release my husband from the burden of fulfilling me in areas where I should be looking to you. Help me to accept him the way he is and not try to change him. I leave any changing that needs to be done in your hands, fully accepting that neither of us is perfect and never will be. Only you, Lord, are perfect and I look to you to perfect us. Teach me how to pray for my husband and make my prayers a true language of love.

KEVIN UPDATE

MONDAY, FEBRUARY 28, 2011, 6:08 P.M.

I have been trying to prepare myself for the cancer to return ever since we came home from Rochester in September. Every time that Kevin hurts or has a new body ache, I thought the worst. Is there a new cell cancer growth on that joint now? Is the neck tumor back? Are his bones getting weak? Does he have another infection? How are his kidneys, etc.?

I felt that I needed to be aware that the cancer could come back. I needed to be on guard. The doctor's told us that it's just a matter of time and it will come back. If not Myeloma, a new type of cancer could grow. I know that the doctors are only human, and they make mistakes too. I also know that God is the one who does miracles and decides if this cancer will return or not.

We did coffee hour at church yesterday. Mary Lou, our pastor's wife, came in and spoke to Kevin. She is always smiling and visits with him whenever she gets a chance. I saw them visiting, and I went over to hear what they were talking about. She turned to me and said that she felt that Kevin was totally healed. There is no cancer. I told her of my doubt and what the doctors had told us. She told me not to think about it returning. I need to have faith that God cured it completely. Have joy in the miracle.

I tried to explain why I wanted to prepare myself. I felt I needed to be strong for Kevin and my family if and when it happens again. I don't want to put myself up for a letdown in the future again. I have had so many letdowns this past year already.

Whenever I thought that Kevin was getting better, complications always came up. I told her "We are all going to die sometime. What about God's will be done? I'm all right with whatever God decides to do because I know he has a reason." I saw some disappointment in Mary Lou that I never saw before.

When we left church, Kevin and I talked about this. We told each other that we are the ones in reality and do feel the need to be on guard for ourselves and our children. We need to be prepared so we can continue to be strong and ready when we get this news. We felt that others were way out there in their faith and are not being realistic.

This topic has consumed my thinking for the last two days. I am struggling to find that faith that Mary Lou said I need. The faith that makes me feel that Kevin is totally cured and the cancer will not return. I came up with the following: Am I disappointing God by preparing myself for the possibility of the cancer to return? I do believe that God will and does cure diseases and illnesses. I also believe that God answers prayers, and as you know, we have proof of that this past year.

Well, say, I believe that the cancer is cured. But, say, God doesn't want to cure this one. What if God wants to use us and this journey for others? Will it weaken my faith in God if he doesn't cure Kevin completely? Will I be angry at God? Will my kids be confused and/or angry too? If I tell people that I believe that Kevin is cured and say it comes back. Will their faith in God be weakened? Will they be confused? Will they be turned away from God? Will I be to blame? I don't know what God wants. I feel that God IS walking with us and his will be done.

Do you know that somebody actually had the nerve to tell me that if Kevin isn't cured completely, it's because he didn't have the faith to receive God's healing power? How could they tell me this? How dare they? People do die you know! Just because someone dies, does this mean that their faith was not there? If the cancer comes back, does this mean that Kevin or I don't have the faith necessary? I don't believe this at all but feel that some will think of this to be the case. Will this damage their faith when and if we are let down?

I have trusted in God for healing. Throughout this entire book, I have written about the miracles that we have witnessed. Miracles that God had performed in our lives. Now that Kevin is home and is healthy, did I forget all of this?

Now, am I going to believe in God just enough to get by? Am I going to *really* believe that my God has killed this cancer? I am searching my heart.

WEDNESDAY, MARCH 2, 2011, 4:28 P.M.

I had my appointment to see the psychiatrist today. I was hoping and praying for some answers to my anxiety and depression. After a ninety-minute consultation, it was decided that they needed to do more testing to complete a treatment plan. At this time, however, they feel that my depression was caused from a chemical imbalance.

Chemical imbalance is one of the side effects of traumatic brain injury. Quitting my last medications certainly didn't help at all with my difficulties either.

When the doctor asked me how I was coping with all of the stresses I have been faced with, I told him that I gave it to the foot of the cross. I told him that I made a plan of action and am diligent in being determined to win. He really didn't have much to say after that, but instructed me on my next step.

There was an evaluation that I took that will help determine if I have a chemical imbalance. It was terribly long and asked so many questions about everything under the sun. Once I completed that, an appointment for June was set up to go over the results. Other than that, this specialist refilled my prescription that my family doctor gave me in January for the anxiety. He said that it really isn't a strong pill, but just enough to take the edge off and seems to help me quite a bit.

SUNDAY, MARCH 6

Before church today, Mary Lou had told me two stories of local women who believed, as me about healing. One woman didn't have this total faith but asked God to forgive her for the doubts she had and asked for help. Just by asking, it was given to her. This totally moved me and had given me hope in finding that faith that I was told of.

I asked God to forgive me for not having faith in his healing power. It says in Matthew 4:23, "Jesus went throughout Galilee, teaching in their synagogues, preaching the good news of the kingdom, and healing every disease and sickness among the people." And in Matthew 10:1, "He called his twelve disciples to him and gave them authority to drive out evil spirits and to heal every disease and sickness."

I had been preparing myself for the cancer to return ever since we got back home. It felt like it was just another waiting game, just not knowing when.

I had been confused about this whole healing thing. I mean people do die and people do get sick. Mary Lou told me that it's plain to see that God wants us to live a long life. Psalm 90:10, "The length of our days is seventy years—or eighty, if we have the strength."

When Kevin was first in the ICU in Abbott in January 2009, I had purchased a Bible study book called *Getting a Grip on the Basics of Health and Healing*. I quit doing it, because I didn't have the faith to believe it. I just picked it up and reread some of the beginning of the book. I guess I'm in a different place in my life now than I was back then because I felt different this time as I read some pages of this book.

It is clear to me that I need to have faith in my God to heal Kevin. In order to share this, I need to truly believe it and will do my best. Am I going to only believe in God a little bit? Am I going to leave him in a box until I need him? Will I believe in God totally?

At this time, I have total faith in my God. I know that he has killed the cancer cells in Kevin. Kevin will live a long and healthy life. We all die of something and it's possible that Kevin will die of cancer when he is a ripe old age. Not now!

Until then, we will try to remember to live life daily to the fullest. When challenges and trials come upon us, we will try to remember what we have learned through this journey.

Prayer is the answer to everything. I pray that you find your healing faith for anything that is happening to you in your life.

Life goes on, and we need to be thankful every morning to be alive. It is easy to forget and take life for granted each day. It's easy to get busy in life and don't prioritize like we should. At times it is forgotten what blessings we have and the promises that we were given. We are not perfect, but we have Gods unconditional love and willingness to help us. The only thing we need to do is open the door and let him in.

Chapter 13

FAMILY MEMBER'S THOUGHTS

THE FOLLOWING WAS TONY'S CONFIRMATION SPEECH THIS PAST SUMMER AND SUMS UP HIS THOUGHTS.

Ever since I was born, I have been going to church. Now that I'm graduated everything is becoming so real. I may never have had a legit occurrence like the people who see God and what not, but I have been raised by loving parents who emphasize belief in God.

Now that I'm off to college at NDSU, I will have more responsibilities. I especially have had and will have more responsibilities due to the condition that my step dad, Kevin, is in. However, I can see God at work in Kevin. No one ever expected him to get cancer, but there are always unwelcome surprises. When Kevin was in the hospital with a tumor, everything became so real. I prayed for him every night and still do today. I do now know that God was listening because one day Kevin had fluid in his lungs, which is very bad, and miraculously within a day, were gone and everything was looking up. I am hoping that the power of the Lord will guide Kevin down the path of recovery and help me make key decisions shaping my future both in college and as a Christian.

I know that everyone, including me, puts God in a box. We don't think of praying for help, support or even thanksgiving like we could. We let him out just when we need him at times of trial. I pray that each one of us lets him out much more in our lives.

STEPHANIE'S STORY

Sitting at home, waiting for the phone call to come from Mom with news about Kevin in December of 2009 was agonizing for me. I was home alone. Kaylee was away at a wrestling meet and I don't remember where Tony was.

While Kevin was in the hospital, I missed him. He was in intensive care, and I was just sad. Kevin wasn't around to see me play basketball and do other things that he would have normally been there for.

After Kevin came home from Abbott, I felt that things were definitely tenser in our home than usual.

In three months, Mom and Kevin would have to go to the Mayo Clinic and I would be living with my dad during that time. I missed Kevin and Mom, but I was only fifteen years old and I didn't know what I could do about it.

The frequent trips to Rochester really helped me and was nice. The best trip is when Kaylee and I were with Kevin alone and he opened his eyes. How exciting this was! This gave all of us hope and joy that Kevin was there with us. He heard us, and he knew we were there.

Kevin made his recovery, and one of the factors I think was the love our family had together.

The three months went by, and the car crash definitely stirred everything up. I was very happy to be with my family again in September.

Usually, they say that these times make families grow stronger, but I didn't feel that way. I felt that by not seeing anybody from my small family, I felt alone with nobody to talk to. I felt that we were all growing further apart because I barely talked to Kaylee. Tony and I really never talk, so that really wasn't any different.

When things were back to normal, and looking up for Kevin, my mom didn't take any of her pills. Things got crazier then. I remember waking up in the middle of the night and hearing my mom talking about leaving. I would hear her crying. Feeling badly, I would try to talk some sense into her but nothing worked.

I decided to move out and live with my dad early March 2011. My mom and Kevin don't understand why this happened. I know they love me, but I needed to do this. I just wasn't happy at Howard Lake anymore.

KAYLEE'S STORY

Most people go through life thinking that they will never have to experience a traumatic illness. I have to admit that I was one of those people. I never heard much about cancer until my dad was diagnosed with it over Christmas break of my junior year. I remember the exact moment of the day when I received the phone call. I was at a wrestling meet in Maple Lake when my stepsister Stephanie said that dad was rushed to the emergency room to get a cat-scan on his neck because he was in so much pain. She told me that they found an orange-sized tumor on the back of his neck and that his C-2 vertebrae was close to being disconnected from his spine, which could have killed him. I was mortified. I didn't know what to do or what to think. I forgot where I was when I was on the phone with her and started balling my eyes out and talking very loudly. When I got off the phone, I came back to reality and realized that I was in a gymnasium packed full of people. There were quite a few people looking at me with concern and knew something was wrong. When I came home that night, I remember staying up and talking with Karen for quite awhile about what was going on. We sat there and cried for a good hour. As the week went on, we found out that my dad was going to have surgery to remove the tumor on Christmas Eve. This was the start to an abnormal Christmas. Tony, Stephanie, and I went to my aunt and uncle's house because Karen stayed with my dad during the surgery and the overnight recovery. It was nice to get away with some family members to try and keep my mind clear of things. Although it didn't work all the time, it was better than us three kids spending Christmas at home by ourselves wondering what's going to happen next.

I didn't do much that Christmas break because I felt a pain deep inside that I had never felt before. I felt as if my dad was dead, even though he wasn't. I would cry myself to sleep almost every night because he is my hero. He means the world to me, more than anyone else in my life.

The best thing to do when you experience something like this is to be comforted by other friends. I am the type of person who always loves to be with my friends, go shopping, go to the movies, or go to a bonfire. I felt no desire to do any of that after I found out this news. I was really quiet at school when we came back from break. I wasn't my obnoxious, outgoing self. I stayed very reserved and acted as though I was alone. When people would ask me about the situation, I acted like nothing even happened and he was fine. I ignored the fact that my dad had cancer and didn't like to talk about it with people. That was one of the worst things I could have done. I kept my emotions bottled up inside and wouldn't talk to anyone about my problems, besides my boyfriend at the time. He didn't know how to react to the situation or what to say to me. I felt like I put him in an awkward situation because nobody truly understands what you are feeling unless they've been in the position.

My dad had to get sedated because he reacted to the medications they gave him. This means that he was in a drug-induced coma. He was nonresponsive and sat there with a bunch of cords coming out of his body. He looked so scary. The first time I saw him like that I began weeping and had to step out of the room. It was so hard to see him like that because he looked so helpless, and my dad is always the strong man in the family. He doesn't like to show weakness. I had a million thoughts racing through my brain. What do I do? Is he ever going to come home? Will my dad ever be the same again? I felt like my whole world was ending. I never realized what I should be doing to keep myself healthy. I needed to talk to people about it, especially God. I began praying a lot; for me, my dad, my family, and others who have cancer. After everything that had happened with my dad, I began to have a new compassion for others. I started hearing more about people with cancer or illnesses and suddenly became interested. I want to do something about these diseases and put an end to them. I told myself that when I'm older, besides my main career, I want to do cancer research. I really enjoy helping others and don't want people to have to experience what my family has gone through.

When dad came home from Abbott, I felt complete again. Even though it was amazing to have him back, it still didn't seem the same to me because he wasn't himself. He looked a lot different, acted different, and didn't talk as much as normal. He wasn't able to go to my softball games. I realized that my life is never going to be the same. I needed to have a new outlook on life and change my attitude. Yes, this is going to be a challenge, but I need to tough it out for my dad and try to make the most of life each day. Live in the now. Don't worry about what is going to happen tomorrow, but live each day as if it were going to be your last. As the weeks started going by, my dad started to become a little bit more normal. He gained some weight back and had the ability to do more activities. I noticed that I had become more of myself again. I took interest in my friends again and was a social butterfly at school. Things were finally starting to look up.

I finished up the school year on good terms. After school was out, my dad and Karen informed me that he would be going down to the Mayo clinic in the beginning of July to have a stem-cell transplant. They said they both would be gone for about six to eight weeks. That definitely shocked me. Tony and I were a little bit nervous to find out that we would stay at the house and manage all of the responsibilities ourselves, and Steph would go to her dad's house. We've been so dependent on our parents our whole lives. I mean yes, we've done work around the house, but we've never managed the full house, plus the animals by ourselves; especially not for that long. I was definitely crushed when I heard this because I don't like having them not at the house. Everything just seems so weird when they're gone.

When July came around, I was in Colorado with my softball team for a tournament. My dad and Karen would be leaving before I returned home, so I left the trip early. I got home the day before they left. We said our good-byes to the parents and they left for Rochester. That day was so hard for me. I was emotionally distraught. As a matter of fact, I was the whole summer while they were gone. I didn't know what to do with myself or my time. I don't remember much of what happened last summer; it all seems like a blur to me. I neglected the fact that my dad was sick and I didn't want to see him in the hospital. I would ignore my friends and never hang out with them. I sat at home, played softball, or hung out with my boyfriend. He was the only person I ever wanted to see. Since my dad was gone and he was the most important person in my life, I needed someone to replace him; that's why I wanted to be with my boyfriend all the time. I felt like he could fix the problem and that I didn't have to worry about anything when I was with him. I was totally wrong. I put him in the worst position because I would talk with him about my feelings and he didn't know what to say. He would just do his best to comfort me and tell me things would be okay. I was an emotional train wreck this whole time. Most nights, I would listen to music before I went to bed and cry myself to sleep. I was so sensitive to everything. I felt like a completely different person. I had such a negative vibe the whole summer and never had the motivation to do anything productive.

I visited my dad a couple times and it would make me feel better that day. It was scary to see him in the hospital and stuff, but it was definitely necessary that I go to visit him. That would make me happy for a couple of days, but then I would go back to my emotionally distraught self. Another breaking point in my summer was when Karen told me my dad was sedated again and he was not doing well at all. We went down to visit him and it was really scary. The doctors told Karen that they didn't think he would live to see another day. That was the hardest thing I think I have ever heard in my life. I didn't know how to take it or how to react to it. It was just crazy thinking about it. I didn't like to think about it, but it was always on my mind. Now, I definitely secluded myself from people. I never wanted to leave the house. I think Tony picked up on this and he would always ask me to hang out with him and his friends. Surprisingly, I would occasionally take him up on the offers. It was good for me to hang out with him and his friends to try and make me not think of dad for once.

We had so many people praying for dad to get better and get out of sedation. God performed miracles. He eventually got out of sedation. This was such an amazing thing to witness. It was like I had life again! I wanted to go see my dad and I actually wanted to start hanging out with people again. My parents finally came home the first week in September. It was the best feeling ever to have them back. I felt comforted when I went to bed at night. There wasn't the feeling of not knowing what could happen next. Things felt normal for me. The only hard part was when he would come to my volleyball games. He had no hair. People didn't even recognize him as my dad. It was really different seeing him like that and I didn't like it at all, but it's better than not having him around.

Now that he's been home, things seem like they did three years ago. When I look at him, I don't see him as sick or having cancer. I feel like he is completely healed of everything. People need to spend time with their family and make sure they get along with each other. You never know what your last words to someone might be, so never leave someone on bad terms. Make sure you tell the people you love that you love them. Make sure to take in every breath of life that you can get. Don't take things for granted and cherish the important things in life. It's the small things in life that will make you happy. Your relationships with other people are going to bring you the most happiness in your life. People are meant to intermingle with other human beings and be dependent upon others. After everything that has happened to me, my advice is to live your life how you want to and take every opportunity that comes along. Have no regrets and live as if it's your last day.

KEVIN'S STORY

I don't remember some of the bad times at the hospitals due to medications.

I had faith all along that God had a plan for me with this cancer or I wouldn't still be here.

I am amazed and thankful for the love and support that our families and communities have shown us.

I am not really interested in reading the details of this journey. I'm not ready to relive the situation I was in. I am aware of the miracle of life that God has granted me.

He has given me a second chance of life and for now the cancer is in remission. I'm glad that Karen was there for me. I maybe don't show it at times, but I love her very much and need her in my life to be by my side.

I have pain daily from my neck surgery and get tired quickly. I am determined to keep up the fight and won't get discouraged. I realize that I had major surgery twice in eight months and it will take time to heal.

Every day, I am thankful to be alive. Life seems to be a little different now. We don't go out and socialize as much as we used to. I am pooped out at the end of the day and we are so much more content to just be here at home together than we were in the past. The kids are growing up and starting new chapters in their lives. I am glad to be around to be a part of this.

There are many others who have health issues. I guess my heart and eyes have opened more than in my past to notice this.

I told Karen that if this book she wrote even helps one person, it's worth it.

KAREN'S SUMMARY

If we had to do this all over again, would we have reacted differently? Would we have made different decisions? Would we have been more prepared for the trip to Rochester?

I think about this from time to time. The kids were in the background, but had dealt with trauma also. As you read from Stephanie, she moved out of the house this past March. Should I have left her at our home place in the summer to be together with Tony and Kaylee? Did we make her feel unloved or unwanted by doing this? Would she still be living at home with us? Should I have asked for a friend to live at the home to act as a parent in our absence? Would this have helped Kaylee feel better or more secure? Would this have made Tony and Kaylee feel uncompetitant in their responsibilities being as they were 17 and 18 years old? Should I have made arrangements for someone to come over weekly to see if they needed anything or to talk about anything? Would this have relieved some stress from Tony?

Could have, would have, should have is unknown. This is all part of life. I put those questions at the foot of the cross and have decided to live life with no regrets.

Isiah 41:13 "For I am the Lord, your God, who takes hold of your right hand and says to you, Do not fear; I will help you."

Chapter 14

IDEAS FOR GIVING

LIST OF IDEAS TO DO FOR SOMEONE IN NEED

The following is a list of additional gifts given to us in time of need. Each one of these gifts was truly appreciated and helpful to us. I hope I didn't miss any of them throughout this book.

Most important of all were all of the prayers that we received.

BBQs and blueberry muffins
Chicken bake
Mexican bake, fruit salad, and brownies
A whole ham so I could divide into smaller meal portions for the kids
Lasagna and garlic bread
Goulash
Enchiladas, chips, and brownies
Chicken and rice dish
KFC chicken, potatoes, and coleslaw
Pizza
Egg bake
Buns
CD for calming and four journals for writing
Gift cards for gas
Money for lunches at the hospital
Cleaning my house
Plowing the snow
Some groceries for us
A few days of dog boarding
Visa gift card

Pumpkin bars and cookies
Chocolate chip cookies
Fruit salad, mini meatloaves
Rides to and back from school a number of times
Turkey slaw and snacks for the hospital
Pork chops with rice
Sausage
Stamps, which I used to mail the thank you cards
Work around the house to fix stuff
Subway gift certificates
Papa Murphy gift certificates
Mrs. Beasley's food pack
Free haircuts
Marketplace gift certificate
Tie blankets
Sweatshirt
Books
Subscription to *Outdoor Canada*
Help in finishing sewing my pillows
Salsa and honey
Sunni's gift certificate
Saving me from my summer mishaps
Fixing my manure spreader
Installing my dishwasher
Help with my outside stuff
Cutting wood
Putting on screen for the porch
A hot dish benefit
Gift of money
Dental services
Repair our deck and porch

CANCER'S COLORS

The following is a list of cancers and the support colors associated with them.

Cancer Awareness Ribbon Colors

All Cancers
Lavender

Bladder Cancer
Yellow

Brain Cancer
Grey

Breast Cancer
Pink

Cervical Cancer
Teal/White

Childhood Cancer
Gold

Colon Cancer
Dark Blue

Esophageal Cancer
Periwinkle

Head & Neck Cancer
Burgundy/Ivory

Kidney Cancer
Orange

Leiomyosarcoma
Purple

Leukemia
Orange

Liver Cancer
Emerald

Lung Cancers
White

Lymphoma
Lime

Melanoma
Black

Multiple Myeloma
Burgundy

Ovarian Cancer
Teal

Pancreatic Cancer
Purple

Prostate Cancer
Light Blue

Sarcoma/Bone Cancer
Yellow

Stomach Cancer
Periwinkle

Testicular Cancer
Orchid

Thyroid Cancer
Teal/Pink/Blue

Uterine Cancer
Peach

Honors Caregivers
Plum

Edwards Brothers, Inc.
Thorofare, NJ USA
September 12, 2011